The Wa
Manual
Survival Guide

MW00488130

Fifth Edition

The Washington Manual® Internship Survival Guide

Fifth Edition

Edited by

Thomas M. Ciesielski, MD
Assistant Professor of Medicine
Division of Medical Education
Washington University School of Medicine
St. Louis, Missouri

Thomas M. De Fer, MD
Professor of Medicine
Division of Medical Education
Washington University School of Medicine
St. Louis, Missouri

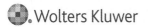 Wolters Kluwer

Philadelphia • Baltimore • New York • London
Buenos Aires • Hong Kong • Sydney • Tokyo

Executive Editor: Rebecca Gaertner
Product Development Editor: Liz Schaeffer
Marketing Manager: Rachel Mante Leung
Senior Production Project Manager: Alicia Jackson
Design Coordinator: Teresa Mallon
Editorial Coordinator: Katie Sharp
Senior Manufacturing Coordinator: Beth Welsh
Prepress Vendor: TNQ Books and Journals

5th edition

Printed in China

Library of Congress Cataloging-in-Publication Data

Names: Ciesielski, Thomas, editor. | De Fer, Thomas M., editor.
Title: The Washington manual internship survival guide / edited by
    Thomas M. Ciesielski, MD, Assistant Professor of Medicine, Division of Medical
    Education, Washington University School of Medicine, St. Louis, Missouri,
    Thomas M. De Fer, MD, Professor of Medicine, Division of Medical Education,
    Washington University School of Medicine, St. Louis, Missouri. Other titles: Manual
    internship survival guide
Description: Fifth edition. | Philadelphia : Wolters Kluwer, [2019] | Revision of: Washington
    manual internship survival guide / written and compiled by Tammy L. Lin, John M. Mohart,
    Kaori A. Sakurai ; executive editor, Thomas M. Defer. c2006. 2nd ed. | Includes bibliographical
    references and index.
Identifiers: LCCN 2018014022 | ISBN 9781975113285 (paperback)
Subjects: LCSH: Internal medicine–Handbooks, manuals, etc. | Interns (Medicine)–
    Handbooks, manuals, etc. | BISAC: MEDICAL / Internal Medicine.
Classification: LCC RC55 .L56 2019 | DDC 616.0078–dc23 LC record available at
    https://lccn.loc.gov/2018014022

RRS1804

Contributing Authors

Asher Albertson, MD
Clinical Fellow
Neurology
Washington University School of
    Medicine
St. Louis, Missouri

Adam Anderson, MD
Assistant Professor
Pulmonary
Washington University School of
    Medicine
St. Louis, Missouri

Rachel Bardowell, MD
Assistant Professor
Division of Hospital Medicine
Washington University School of
    Medicine
St. Louis, Missouri

Kimberly Bartosiak, MD
Resident
Orthopedic Surgery
Washington University School of
    Medicine
St. Louis, Missouri

Sanjeev Bhalla, MD
Professor
Radiology
Washington University School of
    Medicine
St. Louis, Missouri

Neel Bhatt, MD
Resident
Otolaryngology
Washington University School of
    Medicine
St. Louis, Missouri

Martin Boyer, MD
Carol B & Jerome T Loeb Prof of
    Orthopaedic Surgery
Orthopaedic Surgery
Washington University School of
    Medicine
St. Louis, Missouri

Ed Casabar, PharmD
IRB Chair
Human Research Protection
    Office
Washington University School of
    Medicine
St. Louis, Missouri

Steven Cheng, MD
Associate Professor
Nephrology
Washington University School of
    Medicine
St. Louis, Missouri

Collin Chen, MD
Resident
Otolaryngology
Washington University School of
    Medicine
St. Louis, Missouri

Thomas M. Ciesielski, MD
Assistant Professor
Medical Education
Washington University School of
    Medicine
St. Louis, Missouri

Maria Dans, MD
Assistant Professor
Hospitalist Service
Washington University School of
   Medicine
St. Louis, Missouri

Thomas M. De Fer, MD
Professor
Medical Education
Washington University School of
   Medicine
St. Louis, Missouri

Kirsten Dunn, MD
Instructor
Medical Education
Washington University School of
   Medicine
St. Louis, Missouri

Gemma Espejo, MD
Resident
Psychiatry
Washington University School of
   Medicine
St. Louis, Missouri

Kathryn Filson, MD
Resident
Medical Education
Washington University School of
   Medicine
St. Louis, Missouri

Emily Fondahn, MD
Assistant Professor
Medical Education
Washington University School of
   Medicine
St. Louis, Missouri

Matthew Freer, MD
Assistant Professor
Hospital Medicine
Washington University School of
   Medicine
St. Louis, Missouri

Bradley D. Freeman, MD
Professor
Surgery
Washington University School of
   Medicine
St. Louis, Missouri

Jennifer Gross, MD
Resident
Otolaryngology
Washington University School of
   Medicine
St. Louis, Missouri

Thomas Hoyt, MD
Resident
Medical Education
Washington University School of
   Medicine
St. Louis, Missouri

Iris Lee, MD
Resident
Medical Education
Washington University School of
   Medicine
St. Louis, Missouri

Heidi E. L'Esperance, MD
Resident
Otolaryngology
Washington University School of
   Medicine
St. Louis, Missouri

Han Li, MD
Resident
Medical Education
Washington University School of
    Medicine
St. Louis, Missouri

Judith Lieu, MD
Associate Professor
Otolaryngology
Washington University School of
    Medicine
St. Louis, Missouri

Jessica Ma, MD
Instructor
Medical Education
Washington University School of
    Medicine
St. Louis, Missouri

Jared M. McAllister, MD
Research Fellow
Surgery
Washington University School of
    Medicine
St. Louis, Missouri

Zachary Meyer, MD
Resident
Orthopaedic Surgery
Washington University School of
    Medicine
St. Louis, Missouri

Caroline Morris, MD
Resident
Dermatology
Washington University School of
    Medicine
St. Louis, Missouri

Vinaya Mulkareddy, MD
Resident
Medical Education
Washington University School of
    Medicine
St. Louis, Missouri

Brendan O'Connor, MD
Assistant Professor
Psychiatry
Washington University School of
    Medicine
St. Louis, Missouri

David Pham
Instructor
Hospital Medicine
Washington University School of
    Medicine
St. Louis, Missouri

Jane Portell, PharmD
Pharmacist
Drug Information Center
Barnes-Jewish Hospital
St. Louis, Missouri

Samuel Reinhardt, MD
Instructor
Hospital Medicine
Washington University School of
    Medicine
St. Louis, Missouri

Jennifer Riney, PharmD
Pharmacist
Barnes-Jewish Hospital
St. Louis, Missouri

Whitney Ross, MD
Resident
Ob/Gyn Research & Operations
Washington University School of
Medicine
St. Louis, Missouri

Justin Sadhu, MD
Assistant Professor
Cardiovascular Diseases
Washington University School of
Medicine
St. Louis, Missouri

Anup Shetty, MD
Assistant Professor
Radiology
Washington University School of
Medicine
St. Louis, Missouri

Morton Smith, MD
Professor Emeritus
Ophthalmology & Visual Science
Washington University School of
Medicine
St. Louis, Missouri

Tammy Sonn, MD
Associate Professor
Gynecology
Washington University School of
Medicine
St. Louis, Missouri

Kara Sternhell-Blackwell, MD
Associate Professor
Dermatology
Washington University School of
Medicine
St. Louis, Missouri

Renee van Stavern, MD
Professor
Neurology
Washington University School of
Medicine
St. Louis, Missouri

Peter M. Vila, MD
Resident
Otolaryngology
Washington University School of
Medicine
St. Louis, Missouri

Stephanie Velloze, MD
Resident
Medical Education
Washington University School of
Medicine
St. Louis, Missouri

Timothy Yau, MD
Assistant Professor
Nephrology
Washington University School of
Medicine
St. Louis, Missouri

Jennifer Yu, MD
Resident
Surgery
Washington University School of
Medicine
St. Louis, Missouri

Preface

This is the fifth edition of the highly successful, pocket-size, companion survival guide written and edited by former Washington University residents. It is intended to complement the *Washington Manual® of Medical Therapeutics* and the *Washington Manual® of Outpatient Internal Medicine* by providing concise and practical information for those learning the basics of independently practicing clinical medicine. It is written assuming knowledge of pathophysiology and data interpretation. The target audience is primarily those beginning their internship, but this guide may be useful for medical students, residents, and anyone else on the front lines of patient care.

The fifth edition has been updated to be consistent with the most current medical practices. The pace of inpatient medicine requires efficiency and time management skills, especially in our duty-hour regulated environment. In keeping with the concept of a truly pocket-size manual, a very deliberate attempt was made to keep the format succinct so that common workups, cross-cover calls, procedures, and other practical information will always be in a rapidly accessible format. There are also essential cues about "what not to miss" and "when to call for help" for common clinical scenarios. It is also written with the assumption that a standard textbook of internal medicine, the *Washington Manuals®*, a *Sanford Guide, Epocrates*, and Internet access (as well as your resident) are readily available nearby for reference. As with the prior edition, we have included a newly revised rapid-access, pocket-sized card detailing procedural skills and techniques. This card is detachable and can travel with you through the course of your residency and beyond.

Acknowledgments

We wish to thank the Washington University residents and faculty for their enthusiastic support of this project and, even more importantly, their ongoing contributions that have served to make this guide immeasurably better.

We would also like to extend our thanks to Melvin Blanchard, MD, and Vicky Fraser, MD, whose leadership and support have been vital to the continued success of this book. We appreciate the tremendous support of Katie Sharp and Basia Skudrzyk for their coordination of our efforts. From Wolters Kluwer/Lippincott Williams & Wilkins, we are indebted to Rebecca Gaertner and Liz Schaeffer.

T.M.C.
T.M.D.

Contents

Abbreviations List

AAA	Abdominal aortic aneurysm
AMA	Against medical advice
AP	Anteroposterior
APC	Atrial premature contraction
ARF	Acute renal failure
ATN	Acute tubular necrosis
AVNRT	Atrioventricular nodal reentrant tachycardia
AVRT	Atrioventricular reciprocating tachycardia
BBB	Bundle branch block
BP	Bullous pemphigoid
CAD	Coronary artery disease
CHF	Congestive heart failure
COPD	Chronic obstructive pulmonary disease
CPAP	Continuous positive airway pressure
CXR	Chest X-ray
D/C	Discharge
DKA	Diabetic ketoacidosis
ECF	Extracellular fluid
FFP	Fresh frozen plasma
GERD	Gastroesophageal reflux disease
GN	Glomerulonephritis
H&P	History and physical examination
β-hCG	Human chorionic gonadotropin β
Hct	Hematocrit
HEENT	Head, eyes, ears, nose, and throat
HTN	Hypertension
I/O	Input/output
JPCs	Junctional premature contractions
JVP	Jugular venous pressure
LBBB	Left bundle branch block
LMWH	Low-molecular-weight heparin
LP	Lumbar puncture
LVH	Left ventricular hypertrophy
NS	Normal saline
NSAID	Nonsteroidal anti-inflammatory drug
NSR	Normal sinus rhythm
PA	Posteroanterior
PE	Physical examination
PICC	Peripherally inserted central catheter

PID	Pelvic inflammatory disease
PUD	Peptic ulcer disease
PV	Emphigus vulgaris
PVC	Premature ventricular contraction
RR	Respiratory rate
RTA	Renal tubular acidosis
SBO	Small bowel obstruction
SBP	Systolic blood pressure
SJS	Stevens-Johnson syndrome
SOB	Shortness of breath
T	Temperature
TDP	Torsades de pointes
TIA	Transient ischemic attack
TSH	Thyroid-stimulating hormone
TSS	Toxic shock syndrome
UTI	Urinary tract infection
VPC	Ventricular premature contraction

Introduction and Objectives

Thomas M. Ciesielski

INTRODUCTION

Welcome to your intern year. This is a transformative time, and you will likely not forget the first time you walk into a patient's room, whether it's the operating room, emergency room, or hospital ward, and introduce yourself as a physician. It is also a time when you will encounter many new challenges. These will range from very simple to the most complex. You have acquired the tools to address this adversity. Even when you feel most overwhelmed, you are undoubtedly surrounded by a wealth of available resources that include ancillary and nursing staff, fellow interns, senior residents, and attending physicians. As I think back to my intern year, I recall the sage advice from my chief resident, "Intern year is only one year!"

OBJECTIVES

Although the year ahead of you may now seem long and daunting, your tasks are quite achievable. The following rotation objectives were copied from the curriculum for the inpatient general medicine rotation for the internship program at Washington University School of Medicine and Barnes-Jewish Hospital. You can see that not only are the objectives quite simple, but also your rigorous work in medical school has prepared you well to master many of your goals. Your program likely has a similar document, whether in medicine or another specialty. Use these objectives throughout the year as a checklist to remind yourself of your accomplishments and to guide your learning in potential areas of weakness.

* Patient care
  * Gather and synthesize essential and accurate information to define each patient's clinical problems, including performing a thorough history and physical examination.
  * Synthesize data into a prioritized problem list and differential diagnosis, and then develop and achieve comprehensive management plans for patients.

- Manage patients with progressive responsibility and independence.
- Monitor and follow up patients appropriately.
- Know the indications, contraindications, and risks of some invasive procedures and competently perform those invasive procedures.
- Request and provide consultative care.
- Prioritize each day's work (if you're an intern, for yourself; if you're a resident, for your entire team).

- Medical knowledge
  - Demonstrate an increasing fund of knowledge in the range of common problems encountered in inpatient internal medicine and utilize this knowledge in clinical reasoning. If you're a resident, while on service you should become familiar with the diagnostic and therapeutic approach to patients with chest pain, shortness of breath, deep vein thrombosis/pulmonary embolism, nausea/vomiting/diarrhea, fever, mental status changes, abdominal pain, gastrointestinal bleeding, syncope and lightheadedness, renal failure (acute and/or chronic), anemia, hypertension, diabetes mellitus, pneumonia, urinary tract infection, soft tissue infections (e.g., cellulitis, diabetic foot infection, decubitus ulcer), and alcohol withdrawal. You should also demonstrate an increasing ability to teach others on these and other topics.
  - Increase your knowledge of diagnostic testing and procedures.

- Practice-based learning and improvement
  - Understand your limitations of knowledge and judgment, ask for help when needed, and be self-motivated to acquire knowledge.
    - Monitor practice with a goal for improvement.
    - Learn and improve via performance audit.
    - If you are a PGY2 or PGY3, you should learn how to use knowledge of study designs and statistical methods in the critical appraisal of clinical studies and apply to the care of patients.
    - Use information technology to manage information and access online medical information.
  - Accept feedback, learn from your own errors, and develop self-improvement plans.
  - Learn and improve via feedback.
  - Learn and improve at the point of care.

- Interpersonal and communication skills
  - Communicate effectively with patients and caregivers. For example:
    - Demonstrate caring and respectful behaviors with patients, families—including those who are angry and frustrated— and all members of the healthcare team.
    - Counsel and educate patients and their families.
    - Conduct supportive and respectful discussions of code status and advance directives.
  - Communicate effectively with interprofessional teams.
  - Facilitate the learning of students and other healthcare professionals.
  - Ensure appropriate utilization and completion of health records. Demonstrate ability to convey clinical information accurately and concisely in oral presentations and in chart notes.
- Professionalism
  - Display respect, compassion, and integrity.
  - Demonstrate a commitment to excellence and ongoing professional development.
  - Have professional and respectful interactions with patients, caregivers, and members of the interprofessional team.
  - Accept responsibility and follow through on tasks.
  - Develop an appreciation for the ethical, cultural, and socioeconomic dimensions of illness, demonstrating sensitivity and responsiveness to each patient's culture, age, gender, and disabilities.
  - If you are a resident, display initiative and leadership; be able to delegate responsibility appropriately.
  - Exhibit integrity and ethical behavior in professional conduct.
  - Demonstrate a commitment to ethical principles pertaining to provision or withholding of clinical care, confidentiality of patient information, informed consent, and other aspects of clinical care.
- Systems-based practice
  - Work effectively with an interprofessional team (such as with nurses, secretaries, social workers, nutritionists, interpreters, physical and occupational therapists, technicians).
    - If you're a resident, you should develop proficiency in leading the healthcare team and organizing and managing medical care.

- Advocate for quality patient care and assist patients in dealing with system complexities.
- Recognize system errors and advocate for system improvements.
- Identify forces that affect the cost of healthcare and advocate for and practice cost-effective care.
- Transition patients effectively within and across the healthcare delivery system. For example, understand and appreciate the importance of communicating with the primary care physician at the time of admission or soon thereafter.

Keys to Survival

Thomas M. De Fer

1. **DON'T PANIC!** Keep your sense of humor. A positive attitude will take you far.

2. Ask questions and **ASK FOR HELP!** Believe it or not, you are not actually expected to know everything.

3. **TAKE CARE OF YOURSELF.** Sleep when you can, remember to eat, and be mindful of your own health. Don't forget your family and friends.

4. Work hard, stay enthusiastic, and maintain interest. But try not to burn yourself out in the first month.

5. Take care of your patients. You're finally using your expensive education and training. Keep your patients at the center of what you do, and keep their best interests in mind.

6. Be organized and prioritize your tasks. Keep checklists of your tasks and cross them off once you complete. The one with the most checkmarks wins!

7. Verify everything yourself (e.g., lab tests, plain radiographs, ECGs). Any test worth ordering is worth knowing the results of. Never but never make it up! If you don't know, you should say so.

8. Scut happens. Try hard not to leave it to someone else. If you do, they'll return the favor someday.

9. Be kind to the nurses and other ancillary staff. They can make your life much better… or much worse. The choice is mostly yours.

10. When in doubt, go and see the patient!

11. Choose your battles very carefully. Even in the name of patient care, ugly behavior is ugly. You will be remembered for violation. Don't get a reputation!

12. Call for consultations on your patients early in the day and have a specific question you want answered from the consultant.

13. Start thinking about discharge/disposition planning from day 1. Although discharge isn't the goal of all patient care, it should be on your radar screen most of the time.

14. Complete discharge summaries the day the patient leaves.

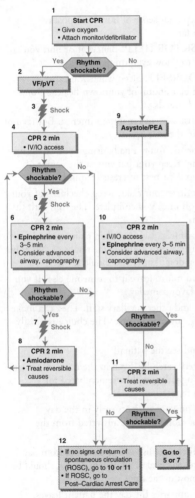

1
Start CPR
• Give oxygen
• Attach monitor/defibrillator

Rhythm shockable? — Yes / No

2
VF/pVT

3 Shock

4
CPR 2 min
• IV/IO access

Rhythm shockable? — No / Yes

5 Shock

6
CPR 2 min
• Epinephrine every 3–5 min
• Consider advanced airway, capnography

Rhythm shockable? — No / Yes

7 Shock

8
CPR 2 min
• Amiodarone
• Treat reversible causes

9
Asystole/PEA

10
CPR 2 min
• IV/IO access
• Epinephrine every 3–5 min
• Consider advanced airway, capnography

Rhythm shockable? — Yes / No

11
CPR 2 min
• Treat reversible causes

Rhythm shockable? — No / Yes

12
• If no signs of return of spontaneous circulation (ROSC), go to **10 or 11**
• If ROSC, go to Post–Cardiac Arrest Care

Go to 5 or 7

CPR Quality

- Push hard (at least 2 inches [5 cm]) and fast (100–120/min) and allow complete chest recoil.
- Minimize interruptions in compressions.
- Avoid excessive ventilation.
- Rotate compressor every 2 minutes, or sooner if fatigued.
- If no advanced airway, 30:2 compression-ventilation ratio.
- Quantitative waveform capnography
  – If PETCO$_2$ <10 mm Hg, attempt to improve CPR quality.
- Intra-arterial pressure
  – If relaxation phase (diastolic) pressure <20 mm Hg, attempt to improve CPR quality.

Shock Energy for Defibrillation

- **Biphasic:** Manufacturer recommendation (eg, initial dose of 120–200 J; if unknown, use maximum available. Second and subsequent doses should be equivalent, and higher doses may be considered.
- **Monophasic:** 360 J

Drug Therapy

- **Epinephrine IV/IO dose:** 1 mg every 3–5 minutes
- **Amiodarone IV/IO dose:** First dose: 300 mg bolus. Second dose: 150 mg.

Advanced Airway

- Endotracheal intubation or supraglottic advanced airway
- Waveform capnography or capnometry to confirm and monitor ET tube placement
- Once advanced airway in place, give 1 breath every 6 seconds (10 breaths/min) with continuous chest compressions

Return of Spontaneous Circulation (ROSC)

- Pulse and blood pressure
- Abrupt sustained increase in PETCO$_2$ (typically ≥40 mm Hg)
- Spontaneous arterial pressure waves with intra-arterial monitoring

Reversible Causes

- **H**ypovolemia
- **H**ypoxia
- **H**ydrogen ion (acidosis)
- **H**ypo-/hyperkalemia
- **H**ypothermia
- **T**ension pneumothorax
- **T**amponade, cardiac
- **T**oxins
- **T**hrombosis, pulmonary
- **T**hrombosis, coronary

Figure 3-1. Adult cardiac arrest algorithm—2015 update. (From American Heart Association. American Heart Association Guidelines for Cardiopulmonary Resuscitation and Emergency Cardiovascular Care. Part 7: Adult Advance Cardiovascular Life Support. Available at: https://eccguidelines.heart.org/index.php/circulation/cpr-ecc-guidelines-2/, with permission (last accessed 2/5/18).)

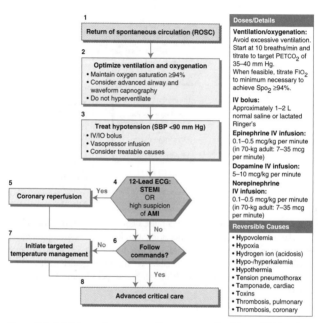

Figure 3-2. Adult immediate post–cardiac arrest care algorithm—2015 update. (From American Heart Association. American Heart Association Guidelines for Cardiopulmonary Resuscitation and Emergency Cardiovascular Care. Part 7: Adult Advance Cardiovascular Life Support. Available at: https://eccguidelines.heart.org/index.php/circulation/cpr-ecc-guidelines-2/, with permission [last accessed 2/5/18].)

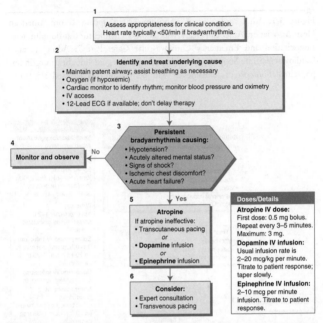

Figure 3-3. Adult bradycardia with a pulse algorithm. (From American Heart Association. American Heart Association Guidelines for Cardiopulmonary Resuscitation and Emergency Cardiovascular Care. Part 7: Adult Advance Cardiovascular Life Support. Available at: https://eccguidelines.heart.org/index.php/circulation/cpr-ecc-guidelines-2/, with permission [last accessed 2/5/18].)

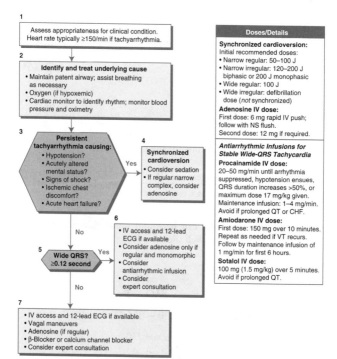

1

Assess appropriateness for clinical condition.
Heart rate typically ≥150/min if tachyarrhythmia.

2

Identify and treat underlying cause
- Maintain patent airway; assist breathing as necessary
- Oxygen (if hypoxemic)
- Cardiac monitor to identify rhythm; monitor blood pressure and oximetry

3

Persistent tachyarrhythmia causing:
- Hypotension?
- Acutely altered mental status?
- Signs of shock?
- Ischemic chest discomfort?
- Acute heart failure?

4

Synchronized cardioversion
- Consider sedation
- If regular narrow complex, consider adenosine

Yes

No

5

Wide QRS?
≥0.12 second

Yes

No

6

- IV access and 12-lead ECG if available
- Consider adenosine only if regular and monomorphic
- Consider antiarrhythmic infusion
- Consider expert consultation

7

- IV access and 12-lead ECG if available
- Vagal maneuvers
- Adenosine (if regular)
- β-Blocker or calcium channel blocker
- Consider expert consultation

Doses/Details

Synchronized cardioversion:
Initial recommended doses:
- Narrow regular: 50–100 J
- Narrow irregular: 120–200 J biphasic or 200 J monophasic
- Wide regular: 100 J
- Wide irregular: defibrillation dose (*not* synchronized)

Adenosine IV dose:
First dose: 6 mg rapid IV push; follow with NS flush.
Second dose: 12 mg if required.

Antiarrhythmic Infusions for Stable Wide-QRS Tachycardia

Procainamide IV dose:
20–50 mg/min until arrhythmia suppressed, hypotension ensues, QRS duration increases >50%, or maximum dose 17 mg/kg given. Maintenance infusion: 1–4 mg/min. Avoid if prolonged QT or CHF.

Amiodarone IV dose:
First dose: 150 mg over 10 minutes. Repeat as needed if VT recurs. Follow by maintenance infusion of 1 mg/min for first 6 hours.

Sotalol IV dose:
100 mg (1.5 mg/kg) over 5 minutes. Avoid if prolonged QT.

Figure 3-4. Adult tachycardia with a pulse algorithm. (From American Heart Association. American Heart Association Guidelines for Cardiopulmonary Resuscitation and Emergency Cardiovascular Care. Part 7: Adult Advance Cardiovascular Life Support. Available at: https://eccguidelines.heart.org/index.php/circulation/cpr-ecc-guidelines-2/, with permission [last accessed 2/5/18].)

Useful Formulae

Thomas M. De Fer

INTRODUCTION

- The most important formula for the intern year:

$$\text{Sleep (h)} = \frac{(\text{discharges} + \text{transfers})}{(\text{admissions} + \text{cross cover})^2} \times \text{number of interns}$$

- Many of these formulae can be found on applications for your electronic devices or on Web sites.

A-a O_2 GRADIENT

$$\text{A-a gradient} = PAO_2 - PaO_2$$

$$PAO_2 = (FiO_2 \times 713) - (PaCO_2/0.8)$$

(all units in mm Hg)

- Estimate for upper limit of normal in room air (in mm Hg) by age (years) = (age/4) + 4.
- Causes of increased A-a gradient: V/Q mismatch, intrapulmonary right-to-left shunt, intracardiac right-to-left shunt, impaired diffusion (room air only)

ANION GAP (SERUM)

$$AG = [Na^+] - ([Cl^-] + [HCO_3^-])$$

(all in mmol/L)

- Normal = 8 to 12 mmol/L
- See Chapter 15, Acid-Base Disorders, for differential diagnosis.

ANION GAP (URINE)

$$UAG = (U_{[Na^+]} + U_{[K^+]}) - U_{[Cl^-]}$$

(all in mmol/L)

- Normal = slightly positive
- UAG is **negative** in diarrhea-induced nongap metabolic acidosis (**enhanced** urinary NH_4^+ excretion).
- UAG is **positive** in distal RTA-induced nongap metabolic acidosis (**impaired** urinary NH_4^+ excretion).
- See Chapter 15, Acid-Base Disorders, for differential diagnosis.

BODY MASS INDEX

$$BMI = wt/(ht)^2$$

(wt in kg, ht in m)

- <18.5 = underweight
- 18.5-24.9 = normal weight
- 25-29.9 = overweight
- >30 = obese
- >40 = morbidly obese

CREATININE CLEARANCE/GLOMERULAR FILTRATION RATE

Estimated (Cockcroft-Gault Formula)

$$CrCl = [(140 - age) \times weight]/[serum\ Cr \times 72] \times 0.85\ (if\ female)$$

(weight in kg, Cr in mg/dL)

Estimated (MDRD)

$$eGFR = 175 \times (SCr)^{-1.54} \times age^{-0.203}$$
$$\times 0.742\ (if\ female)$$
$$\times 1.21\ (if\ black)$$

(eGFR in mL/min per 1.73m², Cr in mg/dL)

- Um, yeah, like you're going to calculate those exponents in your head. Obviously, this is too complicated without a calculator.
- If you care, MDRD stands for Modification of Diet in Renal Disease (study).
- MDRD is fairly accurate for patients with known chronic kidney disease and who are not hospitalized.

Estimated (The Chronic Kidney Disease Epidemiology Collaboration)

$$eGFR = 141 \times \min{(SCr/\kappa, 1)}^{\alpha} \times \max{(SCr/\kappa, 1)}^{-1.209} \times 0.993^{age}$$
$$\times\ 1.018\ (if\ female)$$
$$\times\ 1.159\ (if\ black)$$
$$(eGFR\ in\ mL/min\ per\ 1.73m^2,\ Cr\ in\ mg/dL)$$

- Again, ain't no way anyone can calculate that in his/her head.
- More accurate when GFR is close to normal.

Measured (24-h)

$$CrCl = (U_{[Cr]} \times U_{volume})/(P_{[Cr]} \times 24 \times 60)$$
$$(Cr\ in\ mg/dL,\ volume\ in\ mL,\ and\ time\ in\ min)$$

CORRECTED SERUM CALCIUM

$$Corrected\ serum\ Ca = [Ca^{+2}] + \left[0.8 \times (4.0 - [albumin])\right]$$
$$([Ca^{+2}]\ in\ mg/dL,\ albumin\ in\ g/d)$$

CORRECTED SERUM SODIUM

$$Corrected\ serum\ Na = [Na^+] + \left[0.016 \times ([glucose] - 100)\right]$$
$$([Na^+]\ in\ mmol/L,\ [glucose]\ in\ mg/dL)$$

FRACTIONAL EXCRETION OF SODIUM

$$FE_{Na} = (U_{[Na^+]} \times P_{[Cr]})/(P_{[Na^+]} \times U_{[Cr]}) \times 100$$
$$(U_{[Na^+]}\ and\ P_{[Na^+]}\ in\ mmol/L;\ U_{[Cr]}\ and\ P_{[Cr]}\ in\ mg/dL)$$

- FE_{Na} <1% in prerenal states, early acute tubular necrosis, contrast or heme-pigment nephropathy, and acute glomerulonephritis.
- Not valid when diuretics have been given.
- See "Acute Kidney Injury" section in Chapter 12, Top 10 Workups.

FRACTIONAL EXCRETION OF UREA

$$FE_{urea} = [(U_{[urea]} \times P_{[Cr]})/(P_{[urea]} \times U_{[Cr]})] \times 100$$

(all units in mg/dL)

- FE_{urea} <35% in prerenal states.
- Not affected by diuretics.
- See "Acute Kidney Injury" section in Chapter 12, Top 10 Workups.

MEAN ARTERIAL PRESSURE

$$\text{Mean arterial pressure} = [SBP + (2 \times DBP)]/3$$

MODEL FOR END-STAGE LIVER DISEASE

$$MELD = (3.78 \times Ln[bilirubin]) + (11.2 \times Ln\ INR) + (9.57 \times Ln[SCr]) + 6.43$$

([bilirubin] and [Cr] in mg/dL)

- Who remembers what a nature log is? Rhetorical... Only included to provide the interpretation (Table 4-1).

OSMOLALITY (SERUM, ESTIMATED)

$$\text{Calculated serum osm} = (2 \times [Na^+]) + ([glucose]/18) + ([BUN]/2.8)$$

([Na⁺] in mmol/L; [glucose] and [BUN] in mg/dL)

- To correct for methanol + ([MeOH]/3.2).
- To correct for ethanol + ([EtOH]/4.6).

TABLE 4-1	MORTALITY BASED ON MODEL FOR END-STAGE LIVER DISEASE (MELD) SCORE
MELD Score	Observed Mortality (over 3 mo) (%)
>40	71.3
30-39	52.6
20-29	19.6
10-19	6.0
<9	1.9

Adapted from Wiesner R, et al. Model for end stage liver disease (MELD) and allocation of donor livers. Gastroenterology 2003;124:91-6, with permission.

- To correct for isopropyl alcohol + ([IPA]/6). And in this case, IPA does not stand for India pale ale.
- To correct for ethylene glycol + ([EG]/6.2).
- To correct for mannitol + ([mannitol]/18.2).

OSMOLAL GAP

$$\text{Osmolal gap} = \text{measured } S_{osm} - \text{calculated } S_{osm}$$

- Causes of increased osmolal gap: decreased serum water, hyperproteinemia, hypertriglyceridemia, and presence of unmeasured osmoles (e.g., sorbitol, glycerol, mannitol, ethanol, isopropyl alcohol, acetone, ethyl ether, methanol, and ethylene glycol)
- Every time you drink alcohol you have an osmole gap! Unless you correct for it as mentioned.

RETICULOCYTE INDEX

Reticulocyte index = [reticulocyte count × (Hct/45)]/maturation factor
Maturation factor = 1 + (0.5 × [(45 − Hct)/10])

- Good marrow response = 3.0-6.0. You go marrow!
- Borderline response = 2.0-3.0
- Inadequate response = <2.0. Gosh marrow, is that the best you can do?

MEDICAL EPIDEMIOLOGY

- Yeah, can you believe this stuff actually matters?
- The letters in the following refer to a standard 2 × 2 table presented in Figure 4-1.
- **Sensitivity:** the percentage of patients with the target disease/condition who have a positive result [A/(A + C)]. The greater the sensitivity, the more likely the test will detect patients with the disease. High sensitivity tests are useful clinically to **rule OUT** a disease (SnOUT) (i.e., a negative test result would virtually exclude the possibility of the disease).
- **Specificity:** the percentage of patients without the target disease/condition who have a negative test result [D/(B + D)]. Very specific tests are used to confirm or **rule IN** the presence of disease (SpIN).
- **Positive predictive value:** the percentage of persons with positive test results who actually have the disease/condition [A/(A + B)].
- **Negative predictive value:** the percentage of persons with negative test results in which the disease/condition is absent [D/(C + D)].
- **Number needed to treat:** the number of patients who need to be treated to achieve one additional favorable outcome; calculated as 1/absolute risk reduction, rounded up to the nearest whole number
- **Number needed to harm:** the number of patients who, if they received the experimental treatment, would lead to one additional person being harmed compared with patients who receive the control treatment; calculated as 1/absolute risk increase

Figure 4-1. Medical epidemiology.

	Disease	No disease	
Positive test	True positive (TP) A	False positive (FP) B	All with positive test = A + B Positive predictive value (PPV) = [A/(A + B)]
Negative test	False negative (FN) C	True negative (TN) D	All with negative test = C + D Negative predictive value (NPV) = [D/(C + D)]
	All with disease = A + C Sensitivity = [A/(A + C)]	All without disease = B + D Specificity = [D/(B + D)]	

Patient and Staff Relations

Thomas M. De Fer

WORKING WITH ANCILLARY STAFF

- Give specific directions and use your judgment, but also give others a chance to make suggestions and solve problems. Effectively working with ancillary staff can greatly increase your efficiency and ultimately improve patient care. This is absolutely a team sport!
- Regard ancillary staff as fellow members of the patient care team; they are reaching out to you because of concern for the patient and not to harass you. They have valuable insight that often proves important in patient care.
- A complement for a job well done goes a long way (others are overworked too), and you will be remembered when you need help. When someone performs exemplary work, let his/her supervisor know. Not only that, complementing others improves your overall positive outlook on things. There really are a lot of people around who do the very best job they possibly can every single day.
- Criticize in private. When done, offer only nonjudgmental and constructive feedback. Try to use words that focus on the action rather than the person.
- Efforts to let the team members know the plan can save you phone calls and increase sleep. Your team members will appreciate you for it.

REFERRING A PATIENT

- When referring a patient to the ED or another physician, or transferring a patient, always make a courtesy to call first. Being the recipient of an unannounced patient never feels right.
- Pertinent information includes the following:
  - Who you are
  - Patient identification information
  - Succinct history of the problem
  - Supporting lab data
  - Suggestions for further evaluation

- Likely disposition of the patient
- A contact number where you or someone covering for you can be reached for questions or follow-up information

INTERACTING WITH PATIENTS

- Remember the simple things such as washing your hands, introducing yourself, sitting down, explaining your role, and listening. At the conclusion of an interaction, ask the patient "Is there anything I can do for you while I'm here?"
- Be proactive and address potential concerns, expectations, or questions up front. Checking in with the patient at regular intervals builds rapport and can save you from multiple phone calls. Try to minimize waiting time and interruptions during meetings.
- Be as flexible and as accommodating as you can. Recognize that the patient may be tired of repeating his/her history or having a physical examination. Something as simple as sandwich and some juice can make all the difference in the world.
- Let the patient (and loved ones) know about the management plan at least once a day. Inform them of the test results and changes in the plan, and let them know if consultants will be coming by. If you're ever in doubt as to whether or not you should call a family member about something, you probably should (assuming the patient has OK'd this).
- Avoid promises that you cannot fulfill. This includes the time of discharge or the time of a diagnostic procedure.
- If more than one service is involved, designate someone to be the primary source of communication to avoid confusion.
- A patient's "difficult" behavior may stem from lack of control over decision-making and the situation or lack of insight into his/her medical condition. Past experiences, things the patient may have seen or read in the media, pain, hunger, and fear may all play a role. Some individuals have very different communication styles than your own. Active listening, acknowledging the patient's point of view, and reassurance can go a long way. We are expected to be a congenial as possible, the patient is not. Try this, "It seems that you may be upset. How can I help you?"
- Acknowledge your own frustration and be very mindful of biases. Unintentional misunderstandings can develop on both sides. Seek

the advice of others when necessary. Always try to do what's best for the patient. Set limits when required.

- Potential resource and options for difficult situations are presented in Table 5-1.
- Table 5-2 addresses certain difficult situations. It is important to recall that we can't fix every problem, but we can usually offer some form of advice/assistance. It's also worth noting that sane (i.e., with decision-making capacity) people have the right to make decisions that you would not make. They do it every day of the week.
- Table 5-3 discusses end-of-life issues.

TABLE 5-1	POTENTIAL RESOURCES AND OPTIONS
Resources	**Options**
Nursing supervisor or manager	Individual or joint meetings with or without loved ones (useful for any situation that follows)
Social worker	Initial evaluation discharge plan. This includes nursing home, rehab, or extended care facility placement.
Case coordinator	Return to nursing home issues; durable medical equipment; insurance disputes and concerns.
	Home health/home infusion/hospice referrals
	Transportation issues
Risk management	For litigious patients/family members, if you have concerns about the case, or if you expect a poor outcome
Ombudsman or ethics committee	Helpful if there are disputes between physicians or family members
Family members or loved ones	Proceed cautiously; if the family is in disagreement, try to remain neutral while defending the patient's wishes.
Religious resources	For spiritual support and issues related to death and end of life
A new physician	A new physician may be the best solution if other options have failed. This is rarely necessary.

TABLE 5-2	DEALING WITH DIFFICULT PROBLEMS	
Problems	**Suggestions**	**Potential Actions**
Abuses of the system (i.e., narcotics)	Set boundaries; written agreements are often helpful (be specific in stating the problem and plan).	Notify all members of the team caring for the patient.
		Document concisely in the chart and include on sign out.
Manipulative patients	See previous suggestion.	See previous potential action.
	Coordinate care through one team member to maintain consistency.	
Violent patients (see Chapter 27, Psychiatry)	Safety first.	See previous potential action.
	Tell others you are seeing the patient.	Contact security or law enforcement officials if necessary.
	Try to remain calm and neutral.	Arrange to have security nearby when you see the patient.
	Always stand between the patient and the door.	
	Remove all potentially dangerous items that can be used against you (i.e., stethoscope, necktie).	
Patients who want to leave against medical advice (AMA)	First, establish decisional capacity (see Chapter 27, Psychiatry).	See previous potential action.
	Then, listen to the patient's reason(s).	Have the patient sign AMA form.
	Respond in a nondefensive, nonjudgmental manner.	Carefully document discussion of risks and benefits in the chart.
	Calmly explain the risks and consequences of leaving (if that includes death, say so).	Try to arrange discharge medications and follow-up plans (stating that you'll withhold this as a ploy to convince the patient to stay is inappropriate).
	Explain the benefits of staying and the importance of completing the diagnostic and treatment plan.	Advise the patient to seek medical attention again if condition worsens.
	Be accommodating if possible.	Notify the attending of record of AMA discharge.
	Enlist the help of other team/family members.	

Homelessness or return to abusive situations	Social work is a helpful resource.	Refer patients to local shelters or to local shelters/safe havens. Avoid instructing victims of domestic abuse that they must leave the situation immediately as this can escalate issues). Contact proper authorities (i.e., police, Division of Aging, Child and Family Services).
Refusal of nursing home placement	Social work, family members, and other team members can assist and discuss with the patient. Consider rehabilitation as a potential place for referral.	Careful, neutral documentation in the medical record. Emphasize that it may be a temporary stay. Try to arrange for close outpatient follow-up, home health services, and other family members to check in and help. Ultimately, you may have to respect the patient's wishes.
High likelihood that patient will abuse substances again	Consider chemical dependency consult.	Educate the patient on hazards of substance abuse. Consider inpatient or outpatient follow-up.
Concern for suicide or homicide (see Chapter 27, Psychiatry)	Consider psychiatry consultation; assess competency.	Document carefully in the chart. Place the patient on suicide precautions with a sitter. Consider possible transfer to inpatient psychiatric setting.
Financial difficulties	Social workers or case coordinators can be very helpful.	Notify family members and loved ones. Payment and transportation arrangements can be made. Medication samples. Referral to free clinics and resources. Assistance with applying for Medicaid, disability, etc.

| TABLE 5-3 | ADDRESSING END-OF-LIFE ISSUES |

Issues	Suggestions
Code status Intubation CPR (cardiopulmonary resuscitation) Vasopressors Cardioversion Antibiotics and other medications Nutrition (i.e., G-tubes) Phlebotomy IV lines Withdrawal of support Comfort care	Explain it in the language the patient and family members can understand. Remain neutral, although it is appropriate to give your opinion, especially if asked. Be specific and clear (i.e., the exact interventions to be done or not to be done) in your discussion and **document clearly in the medical record**. **Communicate status with other team members**. Give sufficient time to consider the decision, and explain this decision can be changed (particularly if the circumstances change). Be available for further discussion and questions. If the patient is not able to discuss this with you, contact the primary physician and family members, power of attorney for healthcare decisions, or legal guardian. Do remember that patients with a legal guardian cannot consent to anything.

Patient Safety and Risk Management

6

Jessica Ma and Emily Fondahn

PATIENT SAFETY

- Patient safety is a priority for all healthcare team members.
- Most errors are the result of a faulty system, rather than individual actions, but every healthcare professional remains accountable for his/her choices and actions.
- Safety is improved by learning from errors. It is important to learn how errors can be reported in your institution's event reporting system.
- As an intern, be comfortable speaking up to supervising physicians and staff if you are concerned about an unsafe situation, and seek help if you have questions about patient care.
- See Table 6-1 for the definition of medical errors.

Common Medical Errors

Medication Errors

- Medication errors are the most common errors encountered on the ward and in clinic, and they are the most avoidable. The most common medication errors include missed doses, wrong dosages, infusion errors, patient allergy, and orders entered on the wrong patient.[1]

TABLE 6-1	TYPES OF MEDICAL ERRORS
Type of Error	Explanation
Error	An unintended event or a mistake. An error does not imply outcome
Near miss	An error without a subsequent adverse event due to chance or timely intervention
Bad outcome	An undesirable outcome due to a disease process
Adverse event	A bad outcome due to medical management that could be, but is not necessarily, the result of a mistake or flaw in the system

- High-risk medications can cause significant patient harm if used incorrectly and include oral hypoglycemic agents, insulin, opioids, benzodiazepines, antithrombotic agents, and antiplatelet agents.

tips

- When the patient is unable to provide or recall a list, speak with the outpatient pharmacy or physician to follow up on home medications.
- Ensure that all medications are reconciled, prescriptions are correctly filled out, and the patient has adequate instructions for use, including medication side effects.

Diagnostic Errors

- Diagnostic error occurs when a diagnosis is delayed, missed, or incorrect, and it can occur because of a clinician's cognitive bias. Fatigue, time restraints, and cognitive overloading predispose physicians to cognitive bias.
- *Anchoring bias* is the tendency to rely on the first initial impression as the diagnosis.
- *Framing bias* is when a diagnosis is made because of how the history was presented.

tips

- Do not rely on the history and physical examination done by others.
- If a diagnosis does not fit the patient's clinical picture, take diagnostic time-out by asking yourself:
  - *Was I comprehensive?*
  - *Was my judgment affected by bias?*
  - *What is the worst-case scenario?*
  - *Do I need to make the diagnosis now or can I wait while more information is gathered?*[2]

Procedure-Related Errors

- Errors encountered during procedures include incorrect patient/site; failure to review relevant lab test results, imaging, and medications; surgical site–associated or other healthcare-associated infections; incorrect documentation; poor communication among team members; lack of needed equipment; and retained foreign objects.[3]

- Residents and/or attendings should always be available to help or supervise procedures.

tips

- Obtain informed consent.
- Review pertinent lab test results/imaging, including platelet count and international normalized ratio.
- Mark the procedure site. Review your institution's policies regarding how a procedure site should be marked.
- Conduct a "time-out," which includes at a minimum the patient's identity, procedure site, and the type of procedure set to be done. The time-out should include the immediate members of the procedure team.
- Minimize central line–associated bloodstream infections and any other procedure-related infection using sterile techniques.
- Ensure counts of instruments, sponges, and needles are correct at the end of the procedure.

Transitions of Care

- Handoffs are the process of exchanging patient information and the professional responsibility for caring for a patient. They represent a key area in which important patient information can be lost.
- Verbal and written handoffs should be done at transitions of care, such as change of shift handoffs or discharge from the hospital. Discontinuity of care can lead to unnecessary diagnostic testing or missed diagnostic follow-up care.

tips

- Discharge paperwork should include detailed follow-up diagnostic testing for the patient.
- Follow-up clinic patient notes can include follow-up testing indicated at the next visit.
- Handoffs should detail anticipated events and follow-up testing.

Communication Errors

- Poor communication is a root cause of many patient safety events. An integral part of any admission is open and continued communication with all participants of patient care.

tips

- If there are further questions between consulting services and the primary team, call and speak with the provider for further clarification.
- Prior to the consultation, prepare the question(s) for that subspecialty to answer.
- Be sure to set a comfortable climate in which other healthcare providers can express their opinions and concerns.

Preventing Other Harms

- The intern is often responsible for details in a patient's care that can reduce harm in the hospital.

tip

- A checklist, such as the following, should be reviewed at patient admission, on daily rounds, and at transitions of care. It can be modified for the patient care area.
  - Are isolation precautions needed?
  - What type of venous thromboembolism prophylaxis is needed?
  - Are fall precautions necessary?
  - What is the patient's risk of developing delirium and/or substance withdrawal?
  - What current lines, tubes, and drains (bladder catheter, central line, peripherally inserted catheter) are in place, and are they still a necessity?
  - Are physical or chemical restraints being utilized?
  - What type of pressure ulcer prophylaxis is being employed? Also ensure documentation of any pressure ulcers.

RISK MANAGEMENT

- The goal of risk management is to improve the quality of patient care and reduce the liability to the healthcare provider/system.
- Reporting adverse events not only is important to patient care but also helps identify major system flaws.

When to Call Risk Management

- Unanticipated death
- Permanent harm
- Severe temporary harm and intervention required to sustain life
- An error has been made
- Patient makes threats of litigation
- Any situation that could turn into a legal or risk issue
- Issues with informed consent or patient confidentiality

How to Respond to a Potential Incident

- Arrive as soon as possible. Treat the patient if needed based on the adverse event.
- Document the facts.
- Report injuries.
- Do not state in the medical record that an incident report was completed.

How to Report an Error

- Call risk management at your institution.
- Complete an incident report in your institution's event report system.
- Discuss the situation with your resident and attending as soon as possible.

How to Disclose an Adverse Event

- Errors are bound to occur, and expedient identification, correction, and disclosure can prevent further escalation.
    - Medical errors must be relayed to not only your supervising resident and attending but also charge nurses on the floor and your institution's risk-management department.
    - Physicians are obligated to inform patients when there is an adverse event, even if the patient was not noticeably harmed. Studies have shown that patients are more receptive to open admittance of errors than attempts at concealment.[4]
- Speak with your resident, attending physician, and risk management before disclosing an error.
- Your attending should coordinate disclosure efforts and speak with the patient and family.
- If more than one service is involved, confer and collaborate on the disclosure conversation. The medical care team should deliver a consistent message.

- Give the patient and family an honest, straightforward, and prompt explanation of what occurred.
- Provide an apology for what they are going through.
- If the cause of error is uncertain, do not speculate or hypothesize. State the facts. Tell the patient that further investigation is necessary.
- Identify who will be involved with ongoing care. You may need to transfer the patient's care if the patient-physician relationship has been compromised.
- Tell the patient and family what steps are being undertaken to prevent further error.
- Allow time for questions.
- Speak in layman's terms.
- Be aware of body language.
- Document the discussion with the family including:
  - Time, date, and place
  - Names and relationships of those present
  - Documentation of discussion of event
  - Patient/family response
- Documentation is important whenever there has been an adverse event. Prior to writing a note, give yourself a few minutes to recap what happened. Remember, "If it wasn't documented, it wasn't done."
  - Do's
    - Record changes in patient's condition and response to treatment.
    - Write legibly.
    - Use factual and objective language.
    - Show your thought process.
    - If you consider something potentially serious and rule it out, say so and why.
    - Write plans for future treatment.
    - Chart patient nonadherence.
    - Add addendums when necessary.
  - Don'ts
    - Alter documentation.
    - Use imprecise terms.
    - Write negative comments about the patient, family, or other care providers.
    - Document disputes with other care providers.

Informed Consent

- Informed consent includes the type of procedure, reason or indication for the procedure, benefits and risks of the procedure with disclosure of incidence and severity of complications, and explanation of any alternative procedures.
- Must be obtained from a competent patient, legally appointed guardian, or durable power of attorney for healthcare.
- When a patient is unable to consent, then consent can be obtained from the next of kin, which follows: spouse, adult children, parents, siblings, grandchildren, and grandparents.
- For minors, you must obtain consent of parents or legal guardians. However, minors can consent for themselves if being treated for chemical dependency, sexually transmitted diseases, or pregnancy (excepting elective abortion in some states).
- Two physicians can give consent in a life- or limb-threatening emergency.
- It is important to document informed refusal of a treatment/procedure.

References

1. Medication Errors Patient Safety Primer. AHRQ.gov. 2017. Available at: https://psnet.ahrq.gov/primers/primer/23/medication-errors (last accessed 28/9/17).
2. Ely JW, Graber ML, Croskerry P. Checklists to reduce diagnostic errors. *Acad Med* 2011;86:307-13.
3. Treadwell JR, Lucas S, Tsou AY. Surgical checklists: a systematic review of impacts and implementation. *BMJ Qual Saf* 2014;23:299-318.
4. Robbennolt JK. Apologies and medical error. *Clin Orthop Relat Res* 2009;467:376-82.

Admissions

7

Thomas M. Ciesielski

GENERAL POINTS

- When called with a new admission, obtain the basic demographic information and assess the patient's stability for your service.
  - If it is an admission from the ED, reviewing the chart and vitals and speaking with the physicians can help assess stability. Obtain most recent vital signs, pertinent examination including mental status, key lab data, CXR, ECG, and code status. Review as many lab results and films in the ED as you can.
  - If the patient is admitted directly to the floor (from a clinic or from an outside hospital), it is important to see the patient as soon as possible to assess stability.
- Other helpful tips when calling back the ED include the following:
  - Find out the patient's chief complaints, comorbidities, relevant medical history, and brief current history.
  - Ask what the patient is being admitted for and why the admission is needed. Get the admitting physician's assessment. Ask if the patient is competent, and if he/she wants to be admitted.
  - Confirm IV access.
  - Inquire about major interventions performed, medications given, and consultations pending and determine the necessary follow-up (i.e., lab tests that are pending, consultations that still need to be called, blood transfusions, antibiotics).
  - Find out who the primary physician is and if he/she has been notified.
  - Ask if family members need to be called.
- As you review the available information, determine if this is an appropriate admission for your service (i.e., is there something you can do for the patient that no one else can do or if a different service makes more sense).
- Review old records after confirming stability. Determine when the patient was last admitted and review the chart if possible. **Old records are invaluable**; use them extensively, but always confirm information on your own (trust but verify!).

- After assessing and examining the patient, **complete admission orders as soon as possible.** This helps your nursing colleagues and enables you to get needed lab results in a timely manner. If you need stat labs, always inform the nurses directly. It is also helpful to inform the nurses when your orders are complete.

- Taking a history and performing the physical examination (H&P) should be well engrained by now. It is often helpful to **type or dictate the H&P right after evaluating the patient before moving on to your next admission.**

- If the patient has a private primary care physician, he/she should be notified as soon as possible regarding the admission, and your plan should be communicated to the private physician. **Many private physicians or their covering partners like to be notified as soon as possible**, regardless of the time of day or night.

tips

Remember these three pearls of an admission:

- Assess the stability of the patient immediately.
- Obtain a good H&P, even if this has already been done by another medical team.
- Write orders as soon as possible. This makes the nurses happy and allows you to get the lab data you need to finish your evaluation.

ADMISSION ORDERS

- Many admission diagnoses have preset clinical pathways and associated order sets (i.e., congestive heart failure, asthma), which are often helpful.

- Most teaching hospitals have electronic health records (EHRs) with order sets for admissions. However, if an EHR is not immediately available, the mnemonic ADC VAANDISML may be useful:
  - **A**dmit to ward/attending/house officers
  - **D**iagnosis
  - **C**ondition
  - **V**itals: e.g., routine, every shift, every 2 hours. Always include call orders (e.g., call house officer for systolic blood pressure [SBP] >180 or <90 mm Hg, pulse >130 or <60 bpm, respiratory rate [RR] >30 or <10 breaths per minute, Temperature >38.0°C, O_2 saturation <92%).

- Allergies and reactions
- Activity (ad lib, bed rest with bedside commode, up to chair, etc.)
- Nursing (strict I/O, daily weights, guaiac stools, blood glucose, Foleys, etc.)
- Diet (NPO, prudent diabetic, low fat/low cholesterol, renal, low salt, etc.)
- IV (IV fluids, heplock)
- Special (wound care, consultations with social work, dietitian, and physical therapy/occupational therapy [PT/OT])
- Meds: All medications should include dosage, timing, route, and indications. Don't forget PRN meds or you will be called often; if no contraindications, consider including acetaminophen, bisacodyl, docusate, and aluminum and magnesium hydroxide (Maalox).
- Laboratory (including a.m. labs)
- Don't forget deep venous thrombosis (DVT) prophylaxis for patients at risk of developing a thrombosis and gastrointestinal (GI) prophylaxis for critically ill patients (read further for guidelines)!

Venous Thromboembolism Prophylaxis

- Hospitalized patients usually have at least one risk factor for acquiring a venous thromboembolism (VTE), including DVT and pulmonary embolism.[1] You can assess a patient's risk for developing a venous thromboembolic event using the Padua risk score.[1] **A cumulative score of ≥4 suggests a high risk for developing a VTE.**
  - 3 points: active cancer, previous VTE, reduced mobility ≥3 days, known thrombophilia
  - 2 points: recent trauma or surgery (≤1 mo)
  - 1 point: age ≥70 years, cardiac/respiratory failure, acute myocardial infarction (MI) or ischemic stroke, acute infection and/ or rheumatologic condition, body mass index ≥30, current hormonal treatment
- See Table 7-1 for indications for VTE prophylaxis for medical patients.[1]
- Contraindications to pharmacologic prophylaxis: heparin-induced thrombocytopenia; active bleeding; preoperative within 12 hours or postoperative within 24 hours; lumbar puncture or epidural within 24 hours; recent intraocular or intracranial surgery; coagulopathy
- At Barnes-Jewish Hospital, we primarily use unfractionated heparin (UFH) or low-molecular-weight heparin (LMWH). Your

TABLE 7-1	*CHEST* GUIDELINES FOR VENOUS THROMBOEMBOLISM (VTE) PREVENTIONS[1]
Patients	**Recommendation**
Acutely ill medical patients at increased risk of thrombosis	LMWH, low-dose UFH bid or tid, or fondaparinux[1]
Acutely ill medical patients at low risk of thrombosis	Recommend against the use of pharmacoprophylaxis or mechanical prophylaxis.[1]
Nonorthopedic surgery patients	See 2009 guidelines for VTE prevention in nonorthopedic surgery patients for recommendations, which includes information for surgery type and patient risk.[2]
Orthopedic surgery patients	See 2009 guidelines for VTE prevention in orthopedic surgery patients for recommendations, which includes information on the type of surgery/joint.[3]

LMWH, low-molecular-weight heparin; UFH, unfractionated heparin.

institution may have a different protocol, and it is important to follow your institution's guidelines. For planned invasive procedures (e.g., pacemaker placement, catheterization, surgery), hold UFH 8 hours prior to procedure and LMWH 12 hours prior to procedure!

Gastrointestinal Prophylaxis

- Gastric erosions and stress-induced ulcers can form in critically ill patients. However, not every patient needs GI prophylaxis—if patients do not have any of the risk factors listed here, prophylaxis is not necessary, even in the ICU setting! Most patients will not need GI prophylaxis.

- Risk factors for stress-induced ulcers: mechanical ventilation ≥24 hours, coagulopathy (platelet count <50 000, INR >1.5, dual antiplatelet therapy), history of GI bleed, hypotension requiring vasopressors, sepsis, MI, hepatic failure, acute renal failure, major surgery, ileus, major trauma, severe burns, organ/stem cell transplant, traumatic brain injury, intracranial hemorrhage, spinal cord injury, high-dose corticosteroids, NSAID use (with age >60 years, history of GI bleeding, and/or anticoagulant use).[4]

- At Barnes-Jewish Hospital, we primarily use proton pump inhibitors for stress ulcer prophylaxis. PO is the preferred route, although obviously IV is used if the patient is NPO.

ASSESSMENT/PLAN

- This is the most important part of your note. It is useful to separate this section by problem. The assessment should include a one-line summary of the patient's known medical problems (i.e., hypertension [HTN], type 2 diabetes mellitus [T2DM], coronary artery disease) and those under evaluation (i.e., fever, melena). For example, a 60-year-old woman with a history of HTN, T2DM presents with new-onset chest pain, which is likely cardiac in origin. Include a short differential diagnosis of the current problem.
- The plan should be separated by problem. Cover all problems, including stable issues:
  - Chest pain: No ECG changes, chest pain free now, will rule out MI, monitor on telemetry, continue β-blocker, nitrates, ASA, and ACE-I. NPO for stress thallium in morning assuming rule out of MI.
  - HTN: Good control on current medical regimen.
  - T2DM: Good control with A1C of 6.5%. Continue glucose checks and prudent diabetic diet. Hold PO diabetic meds while NPO. Use insulin sliding scale while NPO.
  - Fluids/electrolytes/nutrition (F/E/N): Monitor I/Os, urine output.
  - Vascular access: Note patient's sites of IV access.
  - Prophylaxis: Indicate plans for DVT prophylaxis and GI prophylaxis if indicated (see previous sections).
  - Disposition: Note any anticipated discharge needs (nursing home placement, home health, home).
  - Code status: Code status should be addressed with every patient admitted regardless of age or disease. Unexpected problems arise too often, and it is better to be prepared.

LABORATORY RESULTS AND ORDERS

It is imperative that orders and lab tests are followed up in a timely manner. You must take personal responsibility to ensure that this is completed.

PATIENT SAFETY ISSUES

Restraints

- Restraints may be needed for patients in a variety of situations. Indications for restraints include the following:
  - Protecting patients from harming themselves (e.g., self-extubation, pulling at Foley catheter, pulling at IV lines)
  - Protecting staff and/or family from patient violence
  - Facilitating medically necessary procedures
  - Preventing disoriented patients from wandering or falling
- Written orders for restraints must include the following:
  - Type of restraint and site (e.g., soft limb restraints on upper extremities, mittens)
  - Start and end times
  - Frequency of monitoring and reevaluation
- The medical reason for restraint use must be clearly documented in the chart. Patients should be reevaluated at least every 24 hours, if not more frequently, and orders renewed if necessary. Consult your hospital policies on this topic for specific information.
- If possible, consider the use of bedside sitters, bed alarms, veil beds, low beds, floor mats, etc., instead of physical restraints. Likewise, chemical restraints (e.g., antipsychotics and low-dose benzodiazepines) should be used only when clearly indicated. Most hospitals have written policies regarding the use of restraints—be sure your orders and documentation comply with hospital policies.

Dangerous Abbreviations for Order Writing

Each hospital may have its own list of unacceptable or dangerous abbreviations. Table 7-2 shows some of the most common ones.[5]

TABLE 7-2   DANGEROUS ABBREVIATIONS

Abbreviation	Intended Meaning	Misinterpretation/Common Error	Correction
U	Units	Mistaken for the numbers "0" or "4" or "cc"	Write "unit"
IU	International units	Mistaken for "IV" or the number "10"	Write "International Units"
Q.D. or Q.O.D	Daily or every other day	Mistaken for each other or QID	Write "Daily"; Write "every other day"
Trailing zero or lack of leading zero	X.0 mg or X mg	Decimal point is missing	Write X mg; Write 0.X mg
MS, MSO, and MgSO	Morphine sulfate or magnesium sulfate	Confused for one another	Write "morphine sulfate"; Write "magnesium sulfate"
µg	Microgram	Mistaken for "mg"	Use "mcg" or "microgram"
AU, AS, AD	Latin abbreviation for both ears, left ear, right ear	Mistaken as the Latin abbreviation "OU" (both eyes); "OS" (left eye); "OD" right eye	Write "both ears"; "left ear"; or "right ear"
cc	Cubic centimeter	Misread as "U" (Units)	Use "mL," "ml," or write out "cubic centimeters" or "milliliters"
HS	Half strength or Latin abbreviation for bedtime	Confused for either half strength or at bedtime. qHS mistaken for every hour.	Write out "half strength" or "at bedtime"
TIW	Three times a week	Misinterpreted as "three times a day" or "twice a week"	Write "three times a week" or specify days (e.g., Q MWF)

From Barnes-Jewish Hospital Department of Pharmacy. St. Louis: Washington University Medical Center, 2010.

References

1. Kahn SR, Lim W, Dunn AS, et al. Prevention of VTE in nonsurgical patients: antithrombotic therapy and prevention of thrombosis, 9th ed: American College of Chest Physicians Evidence-Based Clinical Practice Guidelines. *Chest* 2012;141(2 suppl):e195S-e226S.
2. Gould MK, Garcia DA, Wren SM, et al. Prevention of VTE in nonorthopedic surgical patients: antithrombotic therapy and prevention of thrombosis, 9th ed: American College of Chest Physicians Evidence-Based Clinical Practice Guidelines. *Chest* 2012;141(2 suppl):e227S-e277S.
3. Falck-Ytter Y, Francis CW, Johanson NA, et al. Prevention of VTE in orthopedic surgery patients: antithrombotic therapy and prevention of thrombosis, 9th ed: American College of Chest Physicians Evidence-Based Clinical Practice Guidelines. *Chest* 2012;141(2 suppl):e278S-e325S.
4. BJC Pharmacy and Therapeutics Committee. Stress ulcer prophylaxis. 2013.
5. Barnes-Jewish Hospital Department of Pharmacy. St Louis: Washington University Medical Center, 2010.

Daily Assessments

Thomas M. Ciesielski

ROUNDS

Many programs categorize rounds into prerounds, work rounds, and attending rounds.

Prerounding

- Prerounding is primarily an intern's responsibility.
- Usually allow 30 minutes to an hour before rounds, depending on the number of patients on your service.
- The exact responsibilities should be worked out individually with your resident.
- It is often not necessary to physically see all of your patients before work rounds. However, it is customary to see those patients with an acute problem.
- The most important tasks for prerounding are getting sign-out from the overnight covering physician and catching up on the overnight events. The following example is a good general prerounding plan:
  - Get your sign-out from the night float or cross-cover team. You need to be aware of any major events that happened overnight; this will dictate how you will spend your time prerounding. Check charted vital signs on all your patients. It is also helpful to check nursing and event notes on the computer.
  - Check lab test results and final results of tests (i.e., CXR, echo). Check telemetry every day on all your monitored patients.
  - See the patients. A quick check on your patients (2-3 min per patient) allows you to see how they look and if they have developed any new problems overnight. Of course, patients with more acute illness require more time.

tip

For patients with private physicians, it is often helpful to discuss the plan face-to-face with them in the morning (i.e., try to catch them on their morning rounds). This saves your time in trying to reach them at their offices or in deciphering their progress notes.

DAILY NOTES AND EVALUATION

- Interns are primarily responsible for writing daily notes on each of their patients. The Subjective/Objective/Assessment/Plan (SOAP) format is usually used for daily notes:
  - Subjective: events over the past 24 hours garnered from the patient, cross-covering physician, or nursing staff
  - Objective: factual information, vitals, physical examination, lab test results, lines, and tubes. Include microbiology results, plain radiographs, and other studies here. Always check final official readings of tests.
  - Assessment/Plan: This is the most important part of the note. It is usually categorized by the problem or organ system in the order of importance. Remember to include problems such as electrolyte abnormalities, hypovolemia/hypervolemia, and nutritional status in your problem list and document code status in every note. Also include the type of IV access the patient has and the plan for deep venous thrombosis prophylaxis. In addition, the last category or problem should be discharge planning—including status and goals (e.g., social work arranging placement, home oxygen).
- Medications need to be reviewed daily. Most electronic health records autopopulate medication lists; however, reviewing each medication and dose each day is extremely important. When reviewing the antibiotics, include the number of days each antibiotic has been given and the expected total duration. Similar documentation can be used with other medications that require loading doses or are tapered.
- Review the following items daily:
  - Do IV lines need to be changed?
  - Can IV meds be changed to PO?
  - Can you discontinue the Foley?
  - Do restraint orders need to be renewed?
  - Can you advance the diet and increase the activity of the patient? Is the patient moving his/her bowels? Is there any procedure or test planned that requires that patient to be NPO?
  - PT/OT (physical therapy/occupational therapy) and social work: Are they involved, and should they be? What is the status of discharge planning?
  - Are all meds adjusted for renal or hepatic failure?

- Daily orders should be consolidated and written as early as possible. Don't forget to order a.m. labs for the next morning (only if they are indicated). **Every lab test and study ordered needs to be followed up.**
- If a study needs to be done stat or as soon as possible, notify the nurse directly and consider talking to the radiologist directly. It is helpful to discuss a brief plan with the patient and the nursing staff. This helps them to be part of the team and also helps move things along.

HANDOFFS

Background

- Handoffs have increased since work hour restrictions were put into place.
- Patients cared for by a team other than their primary team are at a higher risk for adverse events. Poor sign-out processes can lead to inefficiencies, delays in care, cost increases, and harm.[1]
- Negative outcomes can be mitigated by formal sign-out systems and curriculum. Medical errors and preventable adverse events decreased after implementation of the IPASS (illness severity, patient summary, action list, situation awareness/contingency planning, and synthesis by receiver) handoff tool.[2]

Necessary Information for Effective Handoff

- Using a standardized format for each patient will make it easy to ensure all necessary information is included in the written handoff.
- For internal medicine trainees at Barnes-Jewish Hospital, our standardized handoff system was adapted from other handoff systems, including a study at three major centers that compiled focus group information from residents on what is required for effective cross-cover.[3] Please see Figure 8-1 for the Barnes-Jewish Hospital standardized handoff template.

Administrative Data

- Patient name, DOB, medical record or hospital number, location
- Code status
- Access
- Acuity (not sick, sick)
- Emergency contact name and phone number

WRITTEN HANDOFF				
Administrative Data		**Background Information**	**To Do**	**Cross Coverage**
Acuity/Access/Code Status/Contact	**Admin Info**			
☐ **Acuity** (assume not sick unless checked) ☐ **Access** ☐ **Code status** ☐ **Emerg contact** (Name and ph #)	☐ Name Team Location DOB MRN	☐ Brief HPI (one liner) ☐ Primary problem ☐ Other active problems ☐ Disposition: location and date if known	Your running to do list	☐ Tasks/tests to follow up on with specific if, then statements ☐ Anticipatory guidance
VERBAL HANDOFF				
☐ Entire team present if possible	☐ Quiet, limit interruptions ☐ Read back critical tasks			☐ Complete one patient at a time

Figure 8-1. Standardized handoff template for internal medicine trainees at Barnes-Jewish Hospital.

Background Data

- Brief HPI (history of present illness) (one-liner)
- Admitting diagnosis/major problem, interventions tried (successful, unsuccessful)
- Other significant problems, interventions tried (successful, unsuccessful)
- Disposition date and location if known

Cross-cover

- Anticipatory guidance with specific if-then statements
- Specific tests ordered that will come back during the coverage period, and what to do with the results

Verbal Communication

- Face-to-face communication between outgoing and oncoming care providers provides additional value.
- Verbally discuss with each patient, tailoring conversation to acuity and complexity of the situation.
- Use read-back techniques for critical tasks.
- Sign-out should preferably occur in a designated location that can allow the physicians caring for the patients to be fully engaged in the process with minimal distraction.

DISCHARGE PLANNING

- Discharge (D/C) planning must be addressed and readdressed constantly. Generally, discharge planning should begin at the time of admission.
- Social work should be consulted on admission if D/C needs are anticipated (assisted living, placement, transportation). Scheduled meetings with case coordinators or social workers are often helpful to reassess the situation and provide updates.
- Orders for physical therapy and occupational therapy should be placed early as well, if deemed appropriate.

References

1. Horwitz LI, Moin T, Krumholz HM, et al. Consequences of inadequate resident sign-out for patient care. *Arch Intern Med* 2008;168:1755-60.
2. Starmer A, Spector ND, Srivastava R, et al. Changes in medical errors after implementation of a handoff program. *N Engl J Med* 2014;371:1803-12.
3. Vidyarthi AR, Arora V, Schnipper JL, et al. Managing discontinuity in academic medical centers: strategies for a safe and effective resident sign out. *J Hosp Med* 2006;1:257-66.

Discharges

9

Thomas M. Ciesielski

INTRODUCTION

- For discharges to be smooth for you and the patient, it requires thinking about discharge early in the hospitalization.
- Prior to discharge, it is critical to ensure your patient has follow-up and has a completely reconciled medication list. In addition, the patient's physician must be aware of any pending issues, studies, or laboratory draws scheduled prior to outpatient follow-up. Communication with all involved parties is crucial to a successful discharge process and ultimately prevents many "bounce backs."
- Significant penalties are in effect for readmissions, and many health systems are focused on preventing readmissions.

DISCHARGE PROCESS/PEARLS

- Obtain social work/case coordinator assistance early in the admission. Try to anticipate issues and problems early on (e.g., transportation, home oxygen, home antibiotics, or nursing/rehabilitation facility placement).
- **Make sure the patient and his/her family are aware of possible discharge dates so that they can arrange their schedules and not be caught off guard.**
- **Arrange for home care services at least 24 hours before discharge** (i.e., home nursing, home laboratory draws, physical therapy, and occupational therapy).
- The Centers for Medicare and Medicaid have criteria for home O_2.[1] Consult with your home institution to ensure patients qualify for home oxygen if needed.
- Discontinue Foley catheters, sitters, telemetry monitoring, and supplemental oxygen as soon as possible. Many rehabilitation facilities require that these are not present 24 hours before discharge.
- Change antibiotics and diuretics to PO the day before discharge. Avoid a.m. lab work the morning of discharge, unless absolutely necessary.

- Provide prescriptions for a 1-month supply of all medications, excluding controlled substances unless absolutely necessary. **Reconcile discharge medications with admission medications. Make a note in the discharge summary of the patient's current medication list as well as any medications that were discontinued or dose-adjusted during the admission.** This paperwork can often be done in advance.

- Dictate or type the discharge summary at the time of discharge. It may seem painful at the time, but it will save you time later and prevent frustration on outpatient follow-up. It is most efficient to complete the document when you are most familiar with the patient and hospital course. Take the extra 5 to 10 minutes to complete it now.

- The hospital course section of a well-organized discharge summary is generally organized by problem list.

DISCHARGE SUMMARY

Each institution has its own rules on discharge summaries. However, most should include the following items:

- Your name, the attending physician's name, and patient name and medical record number

- Date of admission and discharge

- Principal and secondary diagnoses and procedures

- Chief complaint, HPI (history of present illness), and allergies

- Hospital course, including all major events, listing of major radiologic and diagnostic tests and results, and all major therapeutic interventions

- Discharge medications, diet, and activity. Again, make sure to reconcile admission and discharge medications and ensure that your dictated list is correct. Errors in this regard are a major cause of unanticipated outcomes and readmissions.

- Follow-up plans, including dates and times of outpatient appointments/studies

- Condition on discharge

- Copy distribution. Be sure to include any physicians outside your healthcare system who do not have access to your electronic documentation.

Reference

1. Centers for Medicare and Medicaid Services. Home oxygen therapy. 2016. Available at: https://www.cms.gov/Outreach-and-Education/Medicare-Learning-Network-MLN/MLNProducts/Downloads/Home-Oxygen-Therapy-Text-Only.pdf (last accessed 11/2/17).

Cross-coverage

10

Thomas M. Ciesielski

GENERAL POINTS

- At the beginning of your internship, whenever you are called about a patient, go and examine him/her, review the chart, and assess the situation. Discuss your assessment with your resident and determine an appropriate plan. Communicate your impression and plan with the nursing staff and write a brief event note in the chart. Continue to do this until you feel comfortable deciding which situations can be safely handled over the phone.
- **If you have any doubt, see the patient. The patient is always your number-one priority.**
- Once you have seen the patient, write an event note (this can be brief, depending on the situation). Things to document include the following:
    - The reason you were called to see patient (CTSP). For example, CTSP for chest pain.
    - A summary of the situation. This includes the patient's general appearance, vitals, pertinent physical examination, pertinent laboratory, and imaging data.
    - A synopsis of your plan, including all medical decision-making such as diagnostic tests ordered and medications provided
    - Outcome
- A written and verbal handoff is an important component to providing safe cross-coverage of patients (see information on handoffs in Chapter 8, Daily Assessments).

REASONS YOU MUST GO SEE A PATIENT

- Any major changes in clinical status
- Any of the following signs, symptoms, or events:
    - Altered mental status or other changes in neurologic state
    - Dyspnea
    - Chest pain
    - Severe abdominal pain

- Seizures
- Uncontrolled bleeding (hemoptysis, hematemesis, lower gastrointestinal [GI] bleed, hematuria, vaginal bleeding)
- Intractable vomiting
- Severe headache
- New onset of pain
- Falls
- Any major changes in vital signs:
  - Oxygen desaturation
  - Hypotension
  - Arrhythmias (tachyarrhythmias and bradyarrhythmias)
  - Fever associated with changes in mental status, changes in other vital signs

THINGS TO CONSIDER OBTAINING BEFORE ARRIVAL AT BEDSIDE

- **If the nurse's summary of the patient sounds unstable or you are at all unsure, page your resident immediately!**
- It is always appropriate to ask for a full set of vital signs.
- Confirm IV access, or ask your nursing colleagues to begin trying to obtain IV access.
- Oxygen (nasal cannula, face mask), respiratory therapist
- Cardiac monitor, ECG
- Crash/code cart
- Chest radiographs
- Arterial blood gas (ABG) kits
- Blood cultures, if febrile
- Basic lab results, or ask nursing to begin trying to obtain a basic set of lab test results.

APPROPRIATE TRANSFER OF PATIENTS TO THE INTENSIVE CARE UNIT

- If a higher level of care is necessary, it is important to determine which unit is most appropriate for management of the patient. **Your supervising resident should be involved in the decision-making process.**
- Speak to the resident or provider who will be accepting the patient in the ICU to inform him/her of the situation and provide sign-out.

- Have the nursing staff give report to the staff in the unit.
- Write a brief transfer note that includes the following:
  - When and why you were called to see the patient
  - One-line description of patient and his/her comorbidities
  - Your assessment of the situation
  - Your management of the situation, including diagnostic and therapeutic measures, complications, and outcome—include code note, if appropriate
  - Your assessment and plan with brief differential diagnosis for what could be going on
  - Reason for transfer (e.g., hypotension, arrhythmia, unstable vital signs, closer monitoring)
  - Vascular access (e.g., femoral line, peripheral IV)
  - Code status
  - Who has been notified and their contact information (patient's physician, family members)

THINGS THAT CAN WAIT FOR THE PRIMARY TEAM

- Talking to family members; unless urgent, this can usually be handled best by the primary team.
- Major adjustments in medication regimen in a stable patient (i.e., antihypertensive medicines, antibiotics)
- Consultations in nonemergent, stable situations (e.g., GI consult in patient with occult blood-positive brown stool, stable hematocrit, stable vital signs)
- Addressing code status in a stable patient. This is best addressed by the patient's primary medical team who has an established relationship with the patient.

Other Notes of Importance

11

Thomas M. Ciesielski

OFF-SERVICE NOTES

It is your final day on the wards, you've had a grueling month, and the last thing you want to do is write yet another note. However, the presence of concise (going) off-service notes can be a lifesaver to the intern coming onto the service. The essentials include the following items:

- Date of admission
- Any new diagnoses/alterations in previous diagnoses
- Pertinent medical history
- Hospital course (major interventions, events, procedures); this can be organized chronologically or by organ system depending on the patient. This is not a day-by-day recap of every test performed. Distill the story down to its essential details.
- Current medications including day number for antibiotics
- Current pertinent physical examination and lab test results
- Assessment and plan, including goals of care and discharge needs (skilled nursing facility placement, home IV antibiotics, etc.)

PROCEDURE NOTES

These are of vital importance as part of the documentation of the hospital course and should include the following items:

- Procedure and site of procedure. Regulatory bodies now require documentation of a preprocedure "time-out" to confirm the patient's name and the procedure performed. Your electronic health record may have a procedure note template that includes the regulatory compliance pieces, including use of the universal protocol.
- Indication(s)
- Informed consent
- Sterile prep used
- Anesthesia used

48

- Brief description of the procedure
- Specimens and what they were sent for. Of note, any fluids that you just spent your valuable time collecting should be hand delivered to the lab personally.
- Complications
- Postprocedure disposition and pending follow-up studies (e.g., CXR post–central line placement)

DEATH/EXPIRATIONS

Interns are called on quite frequently to pronounce a death. Certain steps must be performed:

- On arrival to the bedside, if family is present, do not forget to comfort the family and offer your condolences—remember they just lost a loved one. You must observe for respirations, auscultate for heart sounds, palpate for a pulse, and attempt to elicit a corneal reflex. Explain to the family members what you are doing. Call an exact time of death that you agree on with the nursing staff.
- Notify your attending physician, the private physician, and family (if not present) immediately, even in the middle of the night. The family must be asked specifically about (1) autopsy, (2) anatomic gift donation, and (3) funeral home. Appropriate forms for an autopsy and anatomic gifts must be completed. Note: Many hospitals have specially trained personnel to handle these particular requests, so be aware that it may not be appropriate for you to approach the family regarding these issues. Notify the appropriate hospital personnel if necessary.
- Complete a death/expiration note or summary. It should include the following information: "Called by nursing to see patient regarding unresponsiveness. The patient was found to be breathless, pulseless, and without heart sounds, blood pressure, and corneal reflexes. The patient was pronounced dead at 9:55 p.m. on August 29, 2017. The patient's private physician and family were notified. The patient's family declined both anatomic gifts and autopsy. The funeral home will be Manchester Mortuary."
- The Certificate of Death must be completed, including your assessment of the cause of death. If the patient has a private physician, the death certificate will likely be completed by the private physician.

Top 10 Workups

12

Vinaya Mulkareddy and Rachel Bardowell

INTRODUCTION

The following are meant to be high-yield approaches to evaluations of common calls and complaints. Several ground rules apply to all changes in clinical status and evaluation of new complaints:

- What are the vital signs? (The ones from right now, not 4 h ago. They are vital, after all.)
- What does the patient look like (sick or not sick)? When in doubt, get thee to the bedside.
- If you need help, ask for it. Medicine is a team sport, and we are all on the patient's team. (On the flip side, when your co-intern or co-resident asks for help, hide in the call room. NO! Pay it forward, of course.)

CHEST PAIN

Ask for an ECG on your way to assess the patient.

Major Causes of Chest Pain

- Cardiovascular: acute coronary syndrome (ACS), acute pericarditis, aortic dissection
- Lungs: pneumonia, pulmonary embolism (PE), pneumothorax
- Gastrointestinal (GI): esophageal spasm, gastroesophageal reflux disease (GERD), peptic ulcer disease (PUD), acute pancreatitis
- Others: costochondritis, herpes zoster, rib fracture, anxiety

Things You Don't Want to Miss (Call Your Resident)

- Myocardial infarction (MI)
- Aortic dissection
- PE
- Pneumothorax

Key History

- Check vitals: blood pressure (BP), pulse, temperature, O_2 saturation, respirations.
- Look at the patient and quickly review the chart.
- Take a focused chest pain history, including quality, duration, radiation, changes with respiration, diaphoresis, and nausea/vomiting (N/V).
- Review ECG and order a troponin.
- If ACS is suspected, give sublingual nitroglycerin and aspirin 325 mg, chewed and nonenteric coated.

Focused Examination

General	Does the patient appear distressed or ill? Do YOU feel distressed or ill?
Vitals	Worrisome findings include hypotension, tachycardia, bradycardia, fever. Take BP in both arms if concerned about aortic dissection. Fever may raise suspicion for PE.
Cardiovascular	Listen for murmurs, rubs, or gallops. Check for chest wall tenderness and any skin lesions. Assess jugular venous pressure (JVP). Check pulses bilaterally in upper and lower extremities, and check for lower extremity edema.
Lungs	Listen for crackles, absent breath sounds on one side, and friction rub.
Abdomen	Examine for distension, tenderness, and bowel sounds.

Laboratory Data and Diagnostic Data

- Obtain an ECG (repeat every 10-15 min as needed; remember that ischemic ECG changes are dynamic) and review telemetry.
- Consider arterial blood gases (ABGs), complete blood count (CBC), basic metabolic panel (BMP), lactate, and troponins (serial, at least 4 h apart).
- Obtain a portable chest radiograph (CXR).
- If you are concerned about a PE, obtain a CT PE protocol (preferred) or ventilation/perfusion (V/Q) scan.
- If you are concerned about aortic dissection, obtain a CT angiogram (dissection protocol) of the chest, abdomen, and pelvis.
- A bedside ultrasound can be useful if the patient exhibits any worrisome signs, to quickly (grossly) evaluate cardiac function and rule out large effusions (does not replace formal echo!). Requires available equipment and some training in ultrasound.

Management

- **ACS** (ST-elevation myocardial infarction [STEMI] or non-ST-elevation myocardial infarction [NSTEMI]/unstable angina)

  - If STEMI (ST elevation of 1 mm or more in two contiguous leads or new left bundle branch block in correct clinical context), call a stat cardiology consult for consideration of **emergent** reperfusion therapy (thrombolytics or percutaneous coronary intervention [PCI]).

  - Ensure the patient is on a cardiac monitor, has IV access, has oxygen (controversial in patients with normal O_2 sat), and has received aspirin.

  - Treat ischemic chest pain with sublingual nitroglycerin and repeat dose q5 minutes × 3 as needed. Monitor for hemodynamic compromise and screen for phosphodiesterase inhibitor use. If there is ongoing pain, consider nitroglycerin IV drip (may cause headache!) or IV morphine 2 mg.

  - Consider β-blocker therapy (e.g., IV metoprolol 5 mg or 25 mg PO), if no hypotension, bradycardia, or acute heart failure (HF), or antiplatelet therapy (e.g., clopidogrel 300 mg PO or ticagrelor 180 mg PO); consider a glycoprotein IIb/IIIa inhibitor for specific patients (obviously with the help of your resident or cardiology fellow), high-potency statin (e.g., atorvastatin 80 mg), anticoagulation with low-molecular-weight heparin (LMWH), or unfractionated heparin (UFH).

  - If NSTEMI/unstable angina, obtain a cardiology consultation for consideration of PCI.

- **Aortic dissection**: Arrange for immediate transfer to the intensive care unit (ICU). Start IV β-blocker (labetalol or esmolol drip) for BP control; nitroprusside can be used if additional BP control is needed. Obtain a stat vascular/thoracic surgery consultation.

- **PE**: Ensure adequate oxygenation; monitor for hemodynamic compromise and administer therapeutic LMWH or UFH. Non–vitamin K antagonist/direct oral anticoagulant (DOAC) therapy may also be initiated.

- **Pneumothorax**: Tension pneumothorax requires immediate needle decompression in the second intercostal space in the midclavicular line, followed by chest tube. Other pneumothoraces involving >20% of the lung or with hemodynamic compromise require a surgery (or interventional pulmonary) consultation for chest tube placement.

- **GI**: Start antacids such as aluminum hydroxide 30 mL PO PRN q4-6h (avoid in patients with renal failure), famotidine 20 mg PO bid, or omeprazole 20 mg PO qday. Elevate the head of the bed, especially after meals.

ABDOMINAL PAIN

Major Causes of Abdominal Pain

Figure 12-1 lists some causes of abdominal pain by location. Generalized abdominal pain may be due to various causes such as appendicitis (at its inception); gastroenteritis or colitis; inflammatory bowel diseases (IBDs) or vasculitis; ischemia; obstruction; peritonitis of any cause; diabetic ketoacidosis; uremia; sickle cell crisis; acute intermittent porphyria; ruptured abdominal aortic aneurysm (AAA); and acute adrenocortical insufficiency.

Things You Don't Want to Miss (Call Your Resident)

- AAA rupture
- Bowel perforation or ischemia
- Ascending cholangitis
- Acute appendicitis
- Retroperitoneal hematoma

Key History

- Check vitals: BP, pulse, respirations, O_2 saturation, and temperature.
- Quickly look at the patient and review the chart.
- Take a focused history, including quality, duration, radiation, changes with respiration/position location, N/V (bilious vs. non-bilious), last bowel movement, and any hematemesis, melena, or hematochezia.
- For women of childbearing age, ask about their last menstrual period.
- Mesenteric ischemia often has pain out of proportion to examination. Consider this, especially in patients with a history of atrial fibrillation (AF) and vascular disease and in elderly patients.

Focused Examination

General	Is the patient distressed or ill-appearing?
Eyes	Check for icterus.
Chest	Check for any skin lesions. Listen for rate and rhythm, murmur, rubs, or gallops. Assess JVP.
Lungs	Listen for crackles, absent breath sounds on one side, and friction rub.

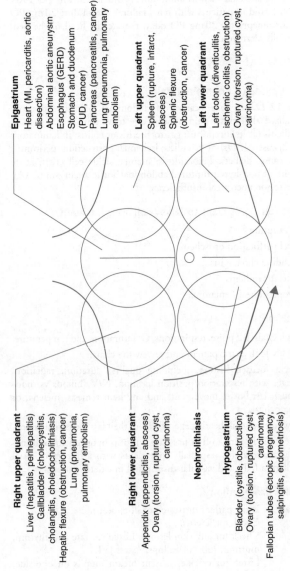

Epigastrium
Heart (MI, pericarditis, aortic dissection)
Abdominal aortic aneurysm
Esophagus (GERD)
Stomach and duodenum (PUD, cancer)
Pancreas (pancreatitis, cancer)
Lung (pneumonia, pulmonary embolism)

Left upper quadrant
Spleen (rupture, infarct, abscess)
Splenic flexure (obstruction, cancer)

Left lower quadrant
Left colon (diverticulitis, ischemic colitis, obstruction)
Ovary (torsion, ruptured cyst, carcinoma)

Right upper quadrant
Liver (hepatitis, perihepatitis)
Gallbladder (cholecystitis, cholangitis, choledocholithiasis)
Hepatic flexure (obstruction, cancer)
Lung (pneumonia, pulmonary embolism)

Right lower quadrant
Appendix (appendicitis, abscess)
Ovary (torsion, ruptured cyst, carcinoma)

Nephrolithiasis

Hypogastrium
Bladder (cystitis, obstruction)
Ovary (torsion, ruptured cyst, carcinoma)
Fallopian tubes (ectopic pregnancy, salpingitis, endometriosis)

Figure 12-1. Major causes of abdominal pain.

Abdomen Auscultate bowel sounds: high-pitched with small bowel obstruction, absent with ileus. Percussion: tympany, shifting dullness. Palpation: guarding, rebound tenderness, Murphy sign, psoas and obturator signs (see Chapter 28, General Surgery). Assess for costovertebral angle tenderness.

Rectal Assess for hemorrhoids and anal fissures. The utility of stool guaiac for occult blood in the inpatient setting is questionable; the appearance of the stool and the presence of gross blood are much more useful.

Pelvic If indicated by history

Laboratory and Diagnostic Data

- Obtain a CBC, complete metabolic panel (CMP), ABG, lactate, amylase, lipase, human chorionic gonadotropin, and urinalysis (UA).
- Films to consider include flat and upright abdominal films, CXR, and ECG. Abdominal CT, ultrasound, or both may be required.

Management

- The initial goal is to determine if the patient has an acute abdomen and needs surgical evaluation and treatment (see Chapter 28, General Surgery).
- Signs and symptoms of an acute abdomen include rebound tenderness or guarding, tachycardia, and hypotension. You can see a low hematocrit (with hemorrhage), elevated white blood cell count, and low bicarbonate.
- Other conditions can be managed using a more detailed approach, after the acute abdomen has been ruled out.
- Keep the patient NPO. Ensure large-bore IV access and run maintenance fluids.

ACUTE ALTERED MENTAL STATUS

- Are the changes acute or subacute? Is the patient confused or is there a change in the level of consciousness? Any recent fall or trauma? Is the patient a diabetic? Does the patient have a cardiac history? Could this be an effect of a prescribed medicine? Could there be an infection? Could this be withdrawal from alcohol or another substance?
- Initial considerations: Think of *TONG* (*T*hiamine, *O*xygen, *N*aloxone, and *G*lucose). Have the nurse obtain a set of vitals and blood glucose.

- **Acute mental status changes require you to see the patient immediately.**

Major Causes of Acute Altered Mental Status

Think *DELIRIUMS*

D = Drug effect or withdrawal (e.g., ethanol, opioids, benzodiazepines, anticholinergics; especially in the elderly, even in low doses)

E = Emotional (e.g., anxiety, pain)

L = Low O_2 (e.g., MI, PE, pneumonia) or high PCO_2 (e.g., chronic obstructive pulmonary disease [COPD])

I = Infection

R = Retention of urine or feces

I = Ictal states

U = Undernutrition/underhydration. OK, somebody just made that up, so the mnemonic would work…

M = Metabolic (electrolytes, glucose, thyroid, liver, kidney)

S = Subdural, acute central nervous system (CNS) processes (e.g., head trauma, hematoma, hydrocephalus, cerebrovascular accident [CVA]/transient ischemic attack [TIA])

Things You Don't Want to Miss (Call Your Resident)

- Sepsis (any etiology) or meningitis
- Intracranial mass or increased intracranial pressure
- Delirium tremens
- Acute CVA
- Neuroleptic malignant syndrome

Key History

- Check BP, pulse, respirations, O_2 saturations, temperature, and blood glucose.
- Quickly look at the patient and review the chart.
- Confirm no falls or trauma.
- Review orders for new medications or opioids.
- Take a focused history from the patient (if possible), including onset and level of responsiveness. Confirm this history with the family or staff.
- Inquire about use of benzodiazepines, alcohol, and illicit substances.

Focused Examination

General	Does the patient appear ill or distressed? Is the patient protecting his/her airway?
Head, eyes, ears, nose, throat (HEENT)	Look for signs of trauma; check pupil size, symmetry, and response to light; evaluate for papilledema and nuchal rigidity.
Chest	Auscultate for murmur, rubs, or gallops.
Lungs	Auscultate for crackles, wheezes, and equal breath sounds.
Abdomen	Assess for ascites, jaundice, and other stigmata of liver disease.
Neurologic	Evaluate for weakness, asterixis, rigidity, or asymmetry. Perform a mental status examination.

Laboratory and Diagnostic Data

- CBC, CMP, ABG, thyroid-stimulating hormone, ammonia level, UA, cultures, ECG, and CXR. Other studies that may be required include lumbar puncture (LP), head imaging (CT/MRI), and electroencephalography.
- Obtain a head CT before LP in the following: elderly, immunocompromised, in the presence of seizures, in those with an altered level of consciousness, and in those with focal neurologic abnormalities.

Management

- Management is based on the findings of examination and laboratory data.
- If meningitis is suspected, LP should be performed as detailed. In addition, empiric antibiotics should be started stat (see Chapter 22, Neurology).
- **If you are worried about a CVA, call neurology immediately!** After all, time is brain (see Chapter 22, Neurology).
- Alcohol withdrawal needs to be treated urgently with benzodiazepines, usually with chlordiazepoxide PO or lorazepam (IV or PO). Thiamine, 100 mg IV/IM, should also be administered, especially before any glucose for encephalopathy prophylaxis. Many institutions use protocols, such as the Clinical Institute Withdrawal Assessment for Alcohol (CIWA), to determine benzodiazepine dose and frequency of assessment.

ACUTE KIDNEY INJURY

- How much of the yellow stuff was produced in the last 24 hours? In the last 8 hours? Does the patient have a Foley catheter inserted? What are the patient's recent electrolytes, especially potassium, blood urea nitrogen (BUN), creatinine, and bicarbonate?
- If the patient has not made any urine, what do you do? If the patient has a Foley, ask the nurse to flush the catheter with 30 mL normal saline (NS). If the patient does not have a Foley catheter, ask the nurse to complete a bladder scan or consider catheter placement. Tell the nurse you will see the patient shortly.

Major Causes of Oliguria

Oliguria is generally defined as <500 mL of urine per 24 hours. Major causes of acute kidney injury (AKI) can be broken down as follows:

- **Prerenal**: volume depletion, HF (a.k.a., cardiorenal), vascular occlusion
- **Renal**: glomerular, tubular/interstitial (acute tubular necrosis [ATN] caused by drugs or toxins), and vascular
- **Postrenal/obstructive**: benign prostatic hypertrophy, clogged Foley catheter, stones

Things You Don't Want to Miss (Call Your Resident)

- Hyperkalemia
- Severe acidosis
- Acute, marked uremia
- Life-threatening volume overload

Key History

- Check vitals: BP, pulse, respirations, O_2 saturations, and temperature. Review BP trend over last 24 to 48 hours if available.
- Quickly see the patient and review the chart.
- Take a focused history, including changes in urination, dysuria, abdominal or flank pain.
- Determine volume status by examining the patient and reviewing ins and outs.
- Check orders and medication list for new medications or possible nephrotoxins (e.g., angiotensin-converting enzyme inhibitors, diuretics, NSAIDs, IV contrast dye, antibiotics).

Focused Examination

General	Does the patient appear sick?
Vitals	Check orthostatics and weight over the past few days.
Cardiovascular	Assess the JVP; listen for a friction rub.
Abdomen	Evaluate for ascites or an enlarged bladder.
Genitourinary (GU)	Consider prostate exam and visual inspection for edema, lesions, bleeding/clots.
Extremities	Assess perfusion, skin turgor; check for edema.
Neurologic	Check for asterixis; assess orientation

Laboratory and Diagnostic Data

- Check BMP.
- UA: Basic dipstick, look at urine sediment for cells, casts, crystals. Yes, actually look under a microscope yourself!
- Check urine electrolytes; calculate the fractional excretion of sodium (FE_{Na}) (and/or FE_{urea} if the patient is on diuretics).
- Consider urine eosinophils, ABG, and ECG (essential if acute hyperkalemia is present).
- Renal ultrasound should be ordered within 24 hours to rule out hydronephrosis and evaluate for evidence of obstruction and chronicity.

Management

- The minimum acceptable urine output is 30 mL/h. If flushing the Foley catheter did not help, ask the nurse to change the Foley catheter. I'm sorry sir, but your urine output is simply unacceptable.
- Initial management should be directed at treating life-threatening electrolyte disorders and correcting volume contraction and hypotension. Obtain diagnostic urinary studies before administration of diuretics. Don't forget to adjust drug doses based on glomerular filtration rate.
- Calculate the FE_{Na}:

$$FE_{Na} = (U_{[Na^+]} \times P_{[Cr]})/(P_{[Na^+]} \times U_{[Cr]}) \times 100$$

This equation is most useful with oliguric renal failure but may be helpful in nonoliguric renal failure.

- $FE_{Na} > 1\%$ to 2% with oliguria is almost always ATN but can be prerenal with diuretics.

- FE_{Na} <1% with oliguria is generally prerenal: volume depletion, severe HF, nephrotic syndrome, NSAID or dye toxicity, sepsis, cyclosporine toxicity, acute glomerulonephritis, and hepatorenal syndrome.
- Calculate FE_{urea} in nonoliguric renal failure or if diuretics have been given. FE_{urea} <35% is consistent with prerenal state.

- If hyperkalemia is suspected, order an ECG and stat whole blood $[K^+]$.
- **A stat renal consultation is required if the patient needs urgent dialysis.**
  - Indications for urgent dialysis include *AEIOU*:

    A = Acidemia (pH <7.2)

    E = Electrolyte disorder (e.g., hyperkalemia when unable to manage medically; see Chapter 14, Fluids and Electrolytes)

    I = Intoxication (e.g., alcohol, salicylates, theophylline, lithium)

    O = Overload (e.g., pulmonary edema when unable to manage medically)

    U = Uremia (encephalopathy, pericarditis)
- **Prerenal causes** can be initially managed with a volume challenge, such as 500 to 1000 mL NS bolus, depending on the cardiovascular status of the patient. This can be followed by NS at a set rate. Specific criteria should be given to the nursing staff (i.e., call if urine output is <30 mL/h). With a fluid challenge, the creatinine level often trends down by the next morning if the cause is prerenal. Alternatively, if HF is suspected, the patient may need diuresis. Urine output and daily weights can be followed and creatinine may improve as volume is removed and hemodynamics improve.
- **Postrenal causes** can be potentially managed by placing a Foley catheter. If immediate flow is obtained, urethral obstruction is likely. If a Foley cannot be placed because of obstruction, consider a urology consultation. They will ask you if you've tried to do it yourself, guaranteed.
- To prevent **contrast-induced nephropathy**, euvolemia is essential. Use 0.45% or 0.9% saline at 1 mg/kg per hour for 6 to 12 hours before and 6 to 12 hours after the procedure. Because of conflicting study results, the use of acetylcysteine remains controversial in most circumstances.

HEADACHE

- How severe is the headache? Has there been a change in consciousness? Are there any new focal CNS symptoms? Has the patient had similar headaches in the past? If so, what precipitates or relieves them?
- **If the headache is severe and acute or associated with N/V, changes in vision, other focal CNS findings, fever, or decreased consciousness, the patient should be seen immediately.** However, you may very well have a headache too, hopefully without any of these findings.

Major Causes and Types of Headache

- Subarachnoid hemorrhage
- Tension
- Migraine
- Cluster
- Medication side effect
- Temporal arteritis
- Infectious (meningitis, sinusitis, fever, in general)
- Trauma
- CVA
- Severe hypertension (HTN)
- Mass lesions

Things You Don't Want to Miss (Call Your Resident)

- Meningitis
- CVA
- Subarachnoid hemorrhage or subdural hematoma
- Mass lesion associated with herniation

Key History

- Check vitals: BP, pulse, respirations, O_2 saturations, and temperature.
- Quickly look at the patient and review the chart.
- A detailed, well-focused history is the best method for evaluating a headache. Most are tension or migraine type, but more serious conditions need to be ruled out.

Focused Examination

General	Does the patient appear ill or distressed?
HEENT	Look for signs of trauma, pupil size, symmetry, response to light, papilledema, nuchal rigidity, temporal artery tenderness, and sinus tenderness.
Neurologic	Thorough examination is mandatory, including mental status.

Laboratory and Diagnostic Data

- Consider CBC and erythrocyte sedimentation rate if temporal arteritis is suspected.
- **Head CT** should be considered for the following:
  - A chronic headache pattern that has changed or a new severe headache occurs
  - A new headache in a patient older than 50 years
  - Focal findings on neurologic examination
- **If meningitis is suspected, an LP should be performed!** Obtain a head CT before LP in the following: elderly, immunocompromised, in the presence of seizures, those with altered level of consciousness, and those with focal neurologic abnormalities (see Chapter 22, Neurology).

Management

- **The initial goal is to exclude the serious life-threatening conditions** mentioned previously. After such conditions have been excluded, management can focus on symptomatic relief.
- For suspected bacterial meningitis, start antibiotics immediately (do not wait for an LP; see Chapter 22, Neurology).
- For suspected subdural hematoma or subarachnoid hemorrhage, obtain CT scan. If positive, a neurosurgery consultation should be obtained.
- Tension headaches and mild migraines can be treated with acetaminophen 650 to 1000 mg PO q6h PRN or ibuprofen 200 to 600 mg PO q6-8h.
- Consider sumatriptan 25 mg PO for moderate to severe migraine headaches; can repeat 25 to 100 mg q2h for maximum of 200 to 300 mg/d. This therapy is most effective when given immediately after the onset of headache. Avoid use in patients with angina or uncontrolled HTN.
- IV ketorolac and prochlorperazine are often used in the hospital for abortive therapy for headache.

ACUTE CHANGES IN BLOOD PRESSURE

This is really a two-for-one, but *Top Eleven Workups* just doesn't have the same ring to it…

HYPOTENSION

- Is the patient unconscious, confused, or lethargic? What has the patient's BP been? What was the reason for admission?
- **Hypotension requires that you see the patient immediately!** Hopefully you didn't need to hear that, but just in case.
- Typically referred to as systolic blood pressure <90 or mean arterial pressure (MAP) <65. Hypotension may also be relative or orthostatic. If impending shock is suspected, ensure adequate IV access (at least 20G IV). Shock is best assessed by looking at end organs: the brain (mental status), heart (chest pain), kidneys (urine output), and skin (cool, clammy); hypotension is also worrisome for shock but not absolutely necessary for diagnosis.

Major Causes of Hypotension

- Cardiogenic
- Hypovolemic
- Distributive (e.g., sepsis, anaphylaxis)
- Obstructive (e.g., acute right HF from PE, cardiac tamponade)

Things You Don't Want to Miss (Call Your Resident)

Shock! Or inadequate organ/tissue perfusion related to circulatory failure. That probably doesn't come as much of a shock to you.

Key History

- Vital signs: Recheck BP (both arms, manually, ensure correct cuff size is used), pulse, respirations, O_2 saturations, and temperature. Repeat often!
- Elevated temperature and hypotension suggest sepsis.
- Quickly assess the patient and review chart. It is important to note the patient's medical comorbidities (e.g., HF, cirrhosis).
- What medications has the patient received recently?
- Has the patient had any volume loss (vomiting/diarrhea) or blood loss?

Focused Examination

General	How distressed or ill does the patient look?
Skin	Note temperature, color, or lack thereof.
Cardiovascular	Check heart rate, JVP, and capillary refill.
Lungs	Listen for breath sounds and crackles on both sides.
GI	Evaluate for any signs of bleeding.
Neurologic	Assess mentation and gross neurologic status.

Laboratory and Diagnostic Data

- Get a lactate, troponins, ECG, ABG, CBC, CMP, and CXR.
- If concern for sepsis, get blood cultures ASAP.
- A bedside cardiac ultrasound evaluation can be helpful if the cause of hypotension is unclear (requires available equipment and specialized training).

Management

- Examine the ECG. A compensatory sinus tachycardia is an expected appropriate response to hypotension. However, ensure that the patient does not have atrial fibrillation, supraventricular tachycardia (SVT), or ventricular tachycardia (VT), which may cause hypotension because of decreased diastolic filling. It's pretty embarrassing to miss VT as a cause of hypotension. Bradycardia may be seen in autonomic dysfunction or heart block.

- Most causes of hypotension require fluids to normalize the intravascular volume, improve preload, and support circulation, and it is the first-line treatment for undifferentiated hypotension. Use 0.9% saline or lactated Ringer's. The exception is cardiogenic shock, which may require preload and afterload reduction, inotropic and/or vasopressor support. **All patients with shock are best managed in the ICU.**

- **Hypovolemic, anaphylactic, and septic shock require fluids.** Fluids, fluids, fluids. Use boluses of 500 to 1000 mL. If no response, repeat bolus or leave fluids open. Give push dose phenylephrine ("Neostick" 0.1-0.5 mg q10-15 min) while setting up a norepinephrine drip if IV fluids fail to improve BP or tissue perfusion.

- **Anaphylactic shock requires epinephrine!** Again, pretty sure you already know that. Give 0.3 mg IM/IV immediately and repeat every 10 to 15 minutes as required. Epinephrine is the most important, but also administer methylprednisolone 125 mg IV and diphenhydramine 25 mg IV. Glucocorticoids take hours to become effective and only prevent prolonged or recurrent anaphylactic reactions. Diphenhydramine is for urticaria/itching. H_2 antihistamines probably add little but are often used.

- **In sepsis, early and aggressive IV fluids and antibiotic administration is the focus of management.** However, continuing hypotension requires ICU admission for vasopressors.
- **Cardiogenic shock** can be the result of an acute MI or worsening HF. However, other causes of hypotension and elevated JVP include (**obstructive shock**) acute cardiac tamponade, PE, and tension pneumothorax. These always need to be considered. If concerned about cardiogenic shock, start dobutamine drip and give furosemide IV. Discontinue β-blockers. Transfer these patients to the cardiac critical care unit as soon as possible.

HYPERTENSION

- What has the patient's BP been? What is the reason for admission? What BP medications has the patient been taking? Does the patient have signs of hypertensive emergency (end-organ damage)?
- The rate of increase of the BP and the setting in which the high BP is occurring are more important than the level of BP itself. Nevertheless, most (but not all!) patients with end-organ damage will have a BP >180/120 mm Hg.
- Very elevated BP alone, in the absence of symptoms or new or progressive end-organ damage, rarely requires aggressive emergent therapy.
- Terminology in this area is not always agreed upon. The term malignant hypertension is no longer used clinically (that doesn't mean there isn't an ICD-10 code for it).
- **So-called hypertensive emergencies require that you see the patient immediately.** This situation may be better termed "severe symptomatic HTN," and it is characterized by end-organ damage directly due to HTN. Prior to your arrival, make sure the patient has an IV and order an ECG.
- **Hypertensive urgencies** are situations of severe **asymptomatic** HTN.

Hypertensive Emergencies

- Encephalopathy
- New papilledema, retinal hemorrhages, exudates
- Intracranial hemorrhage

- Unstable angina or MI
- Acute HF with pulmonary edema
- Aortic dissection
- Eclampsia
- AKI

Things You Don't Want to Miss (Call Your Resident)

Hypertensive emergencies, including all those pesky end-organ damage things

Key History

- Check vitals: BP (both arms, manually, make sure the cuff is of correct size for the patient), pulse, respirations, O_2 saturations, and temperature.
- Quickly look at the patient and review the chart. Get an ECG.
- Ask about localizing symptoms such as chest pain, dyspnea, headache, N/V, visual changes, confusion, and focal neurologic symptoms.

Focused Examination

General	Is the patient distressed or ill-appearing? In many situations the patient will look fine or just a little worried about what all the fuss is about.
HEENT	Check fundi for papilledema, retinal hemorrhages, or exudates. Yes, you ARE expected to do this.
Cardiovascular	Check heart rate, listen for murmurs and gallops, and check JVP and capillary refill.
Lungs	Listen for breath sounds and crackles on both sides.
Neurologic	Look for confusion, evidence of delirium, or focal neurologic deficits.

Laboratory and Diagnostic Data

Consider troponins, ECG, ABG, CBC, BMP, UA, toxicology screen, CXR, head CT or MRI. Obviously, you won't be doing all this on every patient.

Management

- **Treat the patient, not the BP reading. Acute lowering of BP in asymptomatic patients with long-standing HTN can be dangerous.** Resist the urge to do something just to do something.

- Permissive HTN is usually advised by neurologists for patients with an acute ischemic stroke, unless the BP is severely elevated (>220/120 mm Hg) or conditions such as ACS, decompensated HF, dissections, encephalopathy, AKI, and eclampsia coexist. And if this is eclampsia, you darn well better call the OB/GYN!

- Hypertensive emergencies are clearly best treated in an ICU setting. The goal is to reduce the MAP by no more than 25% in the first 2 hours. IV hydralazine, nitroprusside, labetalol, esmolol, clevidipine, and nicardipine are often used. While arranging transfer to the ICU, certain wards allow medications to be started. Consider IV nitroglycerin for HTN associated with MI or pulmonary edema. Labetalol and esmolol are useful in aortic dissection.

- Hypertensive urgencies can usually be managed with oral medications, with the goal of reducing BP over 24 to 48 hours with the MAP not to be lowered more than 25% to 30% in the first few hours. Examples include hydralazine 25 PO, clonidine 0.1 to 0.2 mg PO, or labetalol 200 to 400 mg PO. These can be repeated or titrated every 4 to 8 hours. Close follow-up is essential. Oral and sublingual short-acting nifedipine should not be used because of the risk of rapid drops in BP with compensatory tachycardia and cardiac ischemia.

COMMON ARRHYTHMIAS

- Any chest pain or shortness of breath (SOB)? What is the patient's mental status?
- Review the telemetry or place patient on a cardiac monitor and order a stat ECG. **Patients with chest pain, SOB, altered mental status, or hypotension need to be seen immediately.**

Major Causes of Rapid Heart Rate and Slow Heart Rates

- Rapid rates
  - Regular: sinus tachycardia, SVT, VT, atrial flutter
  - Irregular: atrial fibrillation with rapid ventricular rate (RVR), multifocal atrial tachycardia
- Slow rates
  - Drugs (β-blockers, calcium channel blockers, digoxin)
  - Sick sinus syndrome
  - MI (especially inferior)
  - Atrioventricular (AV) block

Things You Don't Want to Miss (Call Your Resident)

- VT
- Unstable SVT
- High-grade AV block
- ACS

Key History

- Check vitals: BP (hypotension is especially concerning), pulse, respirations, O_2 saturations, and temperature.
- Quickly look at the patient and review the chart, while waiting for a 12-lead ECG.

Focused Examination

General	Does the patient look ill or distressed?
Cardiovascular	Check heart rate and rhythm (regular or irregular?); auscultate for murmurs or gallops; assess JVP, skin temperature/color, and capillary refill.
Lungs	Listen for breath sounds and crackles on both sides.
Neurologic	Evaluate for confusion or change in level of consciousness.

Laboratory and Diagnostic Data

In addition to ECG, consider troponins, ABG, CBC, BMP, Mg, and CXR.

Management

- **Always consider the ABCs first and ensure adequate oxygenation and IV access.** Place the patient on telemetry or a monitor. Consider transfer to a cardiac floor or monitored bed if there is a distinction in your institution.
- **If the patient is hypotensive and has atrial fibrillation with RVR, SVT, or VT, emergency cardioversion may be required.** CLEAR!
  - First, call your resident.
  - If the patient is unstable with serious signs or symptoms, a ventricular rate greater than 150, or both, you should prepare for immediate cardioversion. The patient may require sedation.
  - Serious signs and symptoms per ACLS protocol include chest pain, SOB, decreased level of consciousness, hypotension and shock, congestive HF, and acute MI. Refer to the proper ACLS algorithm at this point (see Chapter 3, ACLS Algorithms).

- **Atrial fibrillation with RVR but without evidence of hemodynamic compromise** can be rate controlled with diltiazem, metoprolol, or esmolol. Amiodarone has a risk of pharmacologic cardioversion, but it is generally considered the best choice if HF and/or an accessory pathway is present.
  - **Diltiazem**: 0.25 mg/kg IVP over 2 minutes; if no response, repeat 0.35 mg/kg IVP over 2 minutes; follow with an IV infusion at 5 to 15 mg/h. Diltiazem is the agent of choice in most patients.
  - **Metoprolol**: 2.5 to 5 mg IVP over 2 minutes every 5 minutes to a total of 15 mg followed by oral dosing. Preferred agent if ischemia is suspected or present.
  - **Esmolol**: 0.5 mg/kg over 1 minute loading dose, followed by 50 μg/kg per minute, maximum 300 μg/kg per minute.
  - **Amiodarone**: 150 mg IV over 10 minutes, followed by infusion of 1 mg/min for 6 hours, and then 0.5 mg/min for 18 hours. Its onset of action is slower than that of calcium channel blockers and β-blockers. Also, be cautious if atrial fibrillation has been present >48 hours, as amiodarone can cause conversion to sinus rhythm and put the patient at risk for cardioembolic stroke.
- **SVT without evidence of hemodynamic compromise** can sometimes be broken with Valsalva maneuver, carotid sinus massage (one side at a time and always listen for bruits first), or both. If still in SVT, try **adenosine**, 6 mg rapid IV push, followed by 12 mg rapid IV push if necessary. Always remember to flush with at least 20 mL of NS after each IV push. If the complex width is narrow with stable BP, diltiazem 10 mg IV or metoprolol 5 mg IVP can be used. Adenosine should be given with significant caution if Wolff-Parkinson-White (WPW) syndrome is suspected.
- For **VT**, if pulseless or without BP, manage as ventricular fibrillation. Call a code for heaven's sake! If VT with serious signs or symptoms, consider immediate synchronized cardioversion. If stable, follow the ACLS protocol (see Chapter 3, ACLS Algorithms).

FEVER

- What was the reason for admission? Is this a new finding? Any associated symptoms (e.g., cough, headache, change in mental status, and N/V)? Any antipyretics or current antibiotics? Any recent surgeries or procedures?
- **Patients with symptoms concerning for meningitis or with hypotension need to be seen immediately.**

Major Causes of Fever

- Infections: Best to think of by site—the lung, urine, IV sites, blood, CNS, abdomen, and pelvis.
- Confirm immune status. **Immunocompromised patients may warrant much more aggressive evaluation and empiric therapy** (e.g., postchemotherapy neutropenic fever).
- Drug-induced fever: Antibiotics and many other drugs have been implicated (e.g., anticonvulsants, allopurinol, heparin).
- Postoperative atelectasis (though often invoked, there is minimal evidence to support this contention)
- Neoplasms
- Rheumatologic diseases
- DVT/PE
- Fever of unknown origin

Things You Don't Want to Miss (Call Your Resident)

- Meningitis
- Septic shock, particularly in neutropenic patients
- Endocarditis
- Serotonin syndrome
- Neuroleptic malignant syndrome

Key History

- Check vitals: BP (hypotension worrisome for septic shock), pulse (tachycardia is expected with fever), respirations (rate may be elevated), O_2 saturations, and temperature.
- Quickly look at the patient and review the chart.

Focused Examination

General	Does the patient appear ill? Check all catheter sites (IV, central line, Foley, G-tube, etc.).
Cardiovascular	Check heart rate, JVP, capillary refill. Any new murmurs?
Lungs	Listen for breath sounds, crackles, wheezes, or rhonchi on both sides.
Abdomen	Assess for localized tenderness and bowel sounds.
Extremities	Check calves for signs of deep venous thrombosis and joints for effusions.
Neurologic	Assess mentation. Look for photophobia, neck stiffness, Brudzinski or Kernig signs.
Skin	Note skin temperature and color; check for rashes.

Laboratory and Diagnostic Data

- Consider CBC, blood cultures (two sets at different sites; if a central line is present, be sure to get one peripheral set as well), CMP, UA and culture, sputum culture and Gram stain, and CXR (PA and lateral if patient can tolerate).
- LP if meningitis is suspected.
- Fluid collections (e.g., pleural effusion, ascites) may need to be sampled.
- Consider *Clostridium difficile* toxin stool testing if patient has watery stools.

Management

- Make sure the patient is hemodynamically stable. Review medications and obtain cultures. Give antipyretics (acetaminophen 650 mg PO/PR or ibuprofen 400 mg PO q6-8h PRN) if patient is symptomatic. Ensure adequate IV access and consider maintenance fluids for insensible losses.
- Consider antibiotics carefully. **If the patient is hemodynamically stable, immunocompetent, not toxic appearing, with no clear source of infection, it may be prudent to withhold antibiotics and await results of cultures and other diagnostic studies.**
- Patients with fever and hypotension require broad-spectrum antibiotics and IV fluids and/or pressors to manage the hypotension. **Septic shock is an emergency** that requires rapid initiation of aggressive therapy (see "Hypotension" section).
- **Patients with fever and meningitis symptoms require antibiotics immediately.** Do not wait for the LP to be completed. Start the antibiotics and then begin the LP.
- Consider changing or removing Foley catheters and any indwelling IV sites.
- Patients with **febrile neutropenia** (absolute neutrophil count [ANC] <1000 cells/mm^3) require a careful physical examination, with particular attention paid to mucosal surfaces, lungs, the skin, and vascular access sites.
  - Blood cultures for bacteria and fungi should be drawn; also consider urine culture, sputum culture, LP, and CXR if clinically indicated.
  - Broad-spectrum antibiotics should be started.
  - Choices for initial therapy include fourth-generation cephalosporin, carbapenem, or an antipseudomonal penicillin, with or without aminoglycoside (i.e., cefepime, meropenem, piperacillin/tazobactam).

- If a catheter-related infection is suspected or the patient is known to be colonized with penicillin-resistant pneumococcus or methicillin-resistant *Staphylococcus aureus*, consider adding vancomycin to the aforementioned regimen.

- What follows is adapted from the Barnes Jewish Hospital Stem Cell Transplant Unit Febrile Neutropenia Pathway. The recommendations are based on antibiotic resistance patterns specific to Barnes Jewish Hospital. **Consult your hospital's antibiogram to tailor antimicrobial therapy to local resistance patterns.**

- Definition of neutropenic fever: temperature ≥38.3°C, or ≥38.0°C for at least 1 hour, with ANC ≤ 500 or anticipate ANC to fall <500.

- Workup: Obtain blood cultures × 2, physical examination, CXR, UA, and culture.

- **Initial treatment**
  - **Cefepime** 1 g IV q8h. *If PCN allergy: aztreonam 2 g IV q8h or ciprofloxacin 400 mg IV q12h.*
  - **Vancomycin** 1 g IV q12h if any of the following are present: severe mucositis, clinical evidence of catheter-related infection, known colonization with resistant *Streptococcus* or *Staphylococcus*, sudden temperature spike >40°C, hypotension, or sepsis.
  - Consider **metronidazole** 500 mg IV q8h, if suspected oropharyngeal or intra-abdominal source.
  - Consider addition of **gentamicin** 5 mg/kg IV q24h × 72 hours, if clinically unstable.
  - Tailor antibiotics based on culture results.

- For patients with persistent fevers or worsening clinical status despite broad-spectrum antibiotics, concern for polymicrobial sepsis or fungal sepsis; consider infectious disease consultation.

- **Duration of antibiotics**
  - Discontinue vancomycin after 72 hours if cultures are negative for coagulase-negative staphylococci, oxacillin-resistant *S. aureus*, cephalosporin-resistant streptococci, or *Corynebacterium jeikeium*.
  - Discontinue double gram-negative rod (GNR) coverage (e.g., aminoglycoside) after 72 hours if cultures are negative for GNR and the patient is clinically stable.

- Culture negative for 3 to 5 days

  If afebrile and ANC ≥500, discontinue after 48 hours.

  If afebrile and ANC <500, continue antibiotics until ANC ≥500 for 48 hours.

  If febrile and ANC ≥500, reassess after 4 to 5 days.

  If febrile and ANC <500, continue antibiotics until neutropenia resolves.

- Culture positive

  Remove line if *Pseudomonas* spp., *Stenotrophomonas maltophilia*, *Acinetobacter* spp., vancomycin-resistant enterococcus, *S. aureus*, *C. jeikeium*, and *Candida* spp.

  For all other organisms and tunneled catheter infections, consider removing line.

  Continue antibiotics until ANC ≥500 for 7 days or for 14 days total, whichever is longer.

- Urinary tract infection: Continue antibiotics until ANC is ≥500.

- Pneumonia

  Bacterial: Until ANC ≥500 for 7 days or for 14 days total, whichever is longer.

  Aspergillus spp. (suspected or proven): Voriconazole (weight-based dosing) and consider infectious disease consultation.

SHORTNESS OF BREATH

- When was the onset of SOB and what was the reason for admission? Does the patient have reactive airway disease or COPD? Is the patient receiving supplemental oxygen?
- Order oxygen and an ABG kit to the bedside. **Patients with SOB need to be seen immediately.**

Major Causes of Shortness of Breath

- Pulmonary: asthma, COPD, PE, pneumonia
- Cardiovascular: HF, ACS/angina, cardiac tamponade
- Others: pneumothorax, obstruction (e.g., mucous plug), anxiety

Things You Don't Want to Miss (Call Your Resident)

- Inadequate tissue oxygenation (i.e., hypoxia)
- Tension pneumothorax
- Airway obstruction

Key History

- Check vitals: BP, pulse, respirations, O_2 saturations, and temperature. Check for a pulsus paradoxus if concern for tamponade.
- Quickly look at the patient and review the chart. Get an ECG, ABG, and CXR if the patient looks sick. Call respiratory therapy for a stat breathing treatment.

Focused Examination

General	Does the patient appear ill or distressed? It is worth noting that SOB often makes patients quite anxious, the nurses and interns as well.
Cardiovascular	Check heart rate; listen for murmurs, rubs, gallops, and distant heart sounds; check JVP, skin temperature/color, and capillary refill.
Lungs	Listen for breath sounds and quality of airflow on both sides. Listen for evidence of consolidation or effusion. Is there wheezing? Crackles? Accessory muscle use?
Neurologic	Assess mentation.

Laboratory and Diagnostic Data

- Consider ABG, ECG, troponins, CBC, D-dimer, CT scan, or V/Q scan, and CXR.
- If you have any doubt at all, get an ABG—if you think about it you should do it. Beware of relying on pulse oximetry alone. It's obvious but worth noting that pulse oximetry tells you nothing about pH or CO_2.
- Bedside lung and cardiac ultrasound can be helpful in the evaluation of the acutely dyspneic patient but requires available equipment and additional training.

Management

- Order empiric oxygen to keep saturations >92%. Be cautious if the patient has COPD and is a retainer of CO_2—in that case, keep O_2 saturations around 88% to 90% and check ABG.
- For asthma (or COPD), administer albuterol (and/or ipratropium) by nebulizer, q2-4h until stable. Consider PO/IV corticosteroids (and antibiotics) depending on severity.
- For HF, is the patient volume overloaded? Raise the head of the patient's bed. Administer IV furosemide and albuterol nebulizer. Remember IV furosemide is twice as strong as PO. Consider morphine or nitroglycerin. Assess for adequate diuresis by monitoring urine output.

- Consider bilevel positive airway pressure for patients with increased work of breathing or hypercarbia, particularly in patients with COPD exacerbations and acute pulmonary edema. Patients requiring the use of noninvasive positive pressure ventilation are best managed in the ICU.
- For suspected cardiac tamponade, order a stat cardiac echo and cardiology consultation.
- For PE, often the patient is tachycardic and tachypneic and has a sudden onset of SOB. The classic ECG findings are S1, Q3, and T3 (S waves in lead I, Q waves in lead III, inverted T waves in lead III) but are often not present. If suspicion is high, consider starting heparin or LMWH prior to obtaining diagnostic imaging. Ensure that the patient has no absolute contraindications to therapeutic anticoagulation. Obtain CT pulmonary angiography or a V/Q scan if renal insufficiency.
- Acute respiratory failure is generally defined by ABG of PO_2 <60 or PCO_2 >50 with a pH <7.3 while on room air. Ensure that the patient hasn't received opioids recently. If so, consider administering naloxone. Acute respiratory acidosis with a pH <7.2 usually requires mechanical ventilation (and ICU transfer).

GASTROINTESTINAL BLEEDING

- When was the onset of bleeding, and what is the reason for admission? Is the bleeding suspicious for an upper (hematemesis, coffee ground emesis, melena) or lower (hematochezia) GI source? How much blood has been lost? It can be remarkably hard to determine this.
- Confirm that the patient has adequate IV access (at least 18G, 2 points of access) and recent CBC and international normalized ratio (INR). Type and cross-match blood. **If the patient is tachycardic or hypotensive, see the patient immediately.**

Major Causes of Gastrointestinal Bleeding

- Upper: esophageal varices, Mallory-Weiss tear, peptic ulcer, esophagitis, neoplasm, aortoenteric fistula (history of AAA repair)
- Lower: diverticulosis, angiodysplasia, neoplasm, IBD, infectious colitis, anorectal disease (hemorrhoids, fissures)

Things You Don't Want to Miss (Call Your Resident)

- Massive hemorrhage leading to hypovolemic shock
- Variceal hemorrhage

- Aortoenteric fistula. Talk about exciting!
- Pretty sure you won't miss these.

Key History

- Check vitals (and repeat often): BP, orthostatic BP (OK, so wouldn't repeat this often), pulse, respirations, O_2 saturations, and temperature.
- Quickly look at the patient and review the chart. Note any history of proceeding emesis, cirrhosis, PUD, recent polypectomy, hypotension/shock, prior surgeries, and radiation.

Focused Examination

General	How distressed or ill does the patient look?
HEENT	Check for conjunctival pallor and scleral icterus.
Cardiovascular	Check heart rate, skin temperature/color, and capillary refill.
Abdomen	Check for tenderness, bowel sounds, and ascites (shifting dullness, bulging flanks, fluid wave).
Rectal	Perform a digital rectal exam and note the color of the stool. Is blood present? Stool guaiac is of limited utility in the inpatient setting with a high level of suspicion for active bleeding.
Neurologic	Evaluate the level of consciousness and ability to protect airway.

Laboratory and Diagnostic Data

- CBC, INR, CMP, and type and screen
- The initial CBC may be deceptive in acute GI bleeding. It will likely need to be repeated. It can take up to 8 hours for CBC to equilibrate, so the initial hematocrit may falsely appear normal or unchanged. In the absence of renal disease, high BUN suggests GI bleeding.

Management

- Insert two large-bore IVs (16G-18G).
- Type and cross-packed red blood cells (RBCs).
- Is the patient receiving anticoagulants or have a significant coagulopathy? If so, stop the anticoagulant and consider reversal/correction with fresh frozen plasma or vitamin K. Target INR of 1.5 and platelets >50K. If the patient is taking dabigatran, reversal with idarucizumab can be accomplished. Other DOACs do not have targeted reversal agents at this time; prothrombin complex

concentrates are currently used for life-threatening hemorrhage. Direct oral anticoagulants have short half-lives, so removing the drug and applying hemostatic and supportive measures are instituted for non-life-threatening bleeds.

- Consider whether special blood products are required on the basis of comorbidities (e.g., irradiated or washed RBCs). Also, consider whether the patient needs premedication with acetaminophen/ diphenhydramine based on prior transfusion reactions.

- Bolster the intravascular volume by giving IV fluids (NS), especially while awaiting blood products. Keep the patient NPO.

- For **upper GI bleeding**, consider insertion of a nasogastric tube and perform lavage to assess if active bleeding is present if this is unclear.

  - Start IV proton pump inhibitor therapy.

  - Obtain GI consultation for endoscopy. If bleeding has stopped and the patient is hemodynamically stable, elective endoscopy can be performed within the next 24 hours. Otherwise, urgent endoscopy may be required for diagnosis and treatment.

  - For active variceal bleeding in patients with cirrhosis, start IV octreotide (somatostatin) at 50 μg bolus, and then 50 μg/h. Start prophylactic IV ceftriaxone 1 g/d, correct coagulation deficits, and replete RBCs as needed. Urgent endoscopy may be required.

- For **lower GI bleeding**, correct fluid status. If hemodynamically stable, obtain GI consultation for colonoscopy. If unstable, an urgent tagged RBC scan should be scheduled. Also, consider CT angiogram or discussion with interventional radiology for embolization.

- Surgery consultation/indications include the following (see Chapter 28, General Surgery):

  - Aortoenteric fistula

  - Uncontrollable or recurrent bleeding

  - Bleeding episode requiring transfusion of more than 6 units of RBCs

  - Visible naked vessel seen in peptic ulcer by endoscopy

  - Bleeding mass/neoplasm

Pain Control

13

Kathryn Filson and Maria Dans

GENERAL PRINCIPLES

- Many complex biopsychosocial factors influence the outward manifestations of pain, both acute and chronic. As a result, pain assessment is subjective; there is no such thing as an objective "pain-o-meter." We must rely on patient description.
- In the hospital, pain rating scales (e.g., "1-10 pain scale" or the "Wong-Baker FACES Pain Rating Scale[1]") are frequently used to standardize these descriptions. Pain rating scales have poor interrater reliability but good intrarater reliability, so they may be helpful for tracking changes in a patient's pain.
- The pain management strategy should be appropriate to the degree of pain and should be put into place concurrently with attempts to diagnose and treat the source of the pain. A pain management strategy based on treating cancer-related pain is outlined in Table 13-1.[2,3]
- While acute pain is often undertreated, complete absence of pain is often an unrealistic goal.
- Patients should be frequently reassessed during analgesic treatment.
- Scheduled analgesics are often more effective than PRN administration.
- Chronic pain is generally defined as pain that last >3 months or past the time of normal tissue healing.
- For chronic pain, long-acting pain medications can improve adherence and reduce some side effects and can be coupled with immediate-release pain analgesics for breakthrough pain at doses of 5% to 15% of the total daily dose.
- General treatment categories for chronic pain include pharmacologic, physical medicine (e.g., physical therapy or occupational therapy), behavioral medicine (e.g., cognitive behavioral therapy), neuromodulation (e.g., transcutaneous electrical nerve stimulation, spinal cord stimulation), interventional (nerve block, ablative techniques), and surgical approaches.

TABLE 13-1	SELECTED AGENTS IN THE THREE-STEP ANALGESIC LADDER[2,3]	
Agent	**Oral**	**Parenteral**
Step 1. Mild pain: nonopioid (and/or adjuvant)		
Acetaminophen	650 mg q4-6h PRN or 1000 mg q6h PRN (max: 4 g/d, 2 g/d if liver disease)	1000 mg IV q6h PRN
Aspirin	325-650 mg q4-6h PRN	–
Ibuprofen	200-800 mg q6-8h PRN	–
Ketorolac	10 mg q4-6h PRN (max: 40 mg/d)	30-60 mg IM or 15-30 mg IV × 1; 15-30 IM/IV q6h PRN; combined PO/IM/IV not to exceed 5 d
Lidocaine patch	5%, 1 transdermal patch to be worn over affected site in 12 h intervals (do not place over rashes or broken skin)	
Gabapentin (for neuropathic pain)[a]	Starting dose 300 mg qhs, titrating to a max of 3600 mg/d divided q8h	–
Pregabalin	100-600 mg/d, divided into 2-3 doses	–
Serotinin and norepineph-rine reuptake inhibitors (SNRIs) (duloxetine, venlafaxine)	Duloxetine: 30 mg PO qday × 1 wk then increase to 60 mg PO qday Venlafaxine: 37.5-225 mg PO qday	
Step 2. Moderate pain: opioid formulated for mild/moderate pain (and/or nonopioid, and/or adjuvant)		
Tramadol	25-100 mg q4-6h (max: 400 mg/d)	–
Hydrocodone/ acetaminophen 5/325 mg (e.g., Vicodin, Norco, Lorcet)[b]	1-2 tablets q4-6h PRN	–

TABLE 13-1	SELECTED AGENTS IN THE THREE-STEP ANALGESIC LADDER[2,3]—cont'd	
Agent	**Oral**	**Parenteral**
Oxycodone/acetaminophen 5/325 mg (e.g., Percocet, Tylox, Roxicet)[b]	1-2 tablets q4-6h PRN	–
Step 3. Severe pain: opioid formulated for moderate/severe pain (and/or nonopioid, and/or adjuvant)		
Morphine	Immediate-release tablets, 10-30 mg q2-4h PRN[c,d] Suppository, 10-20 mg q4h PRN	2-10 mg SC/IM/IV q2-6h PRN
Morphine, extended release (e.g., MS Contin, Oramorph SR)[e]	15 mg q8-12h	–
Hydromorphone	2-4 mg q3-4h PRN	0.5-4 mg SC/IM/IV q3-6h PRN[f]
Fentanyl		Transdermal, 12.5-100 µg/h[e] 50-100 µg IV q1-2h[g]

[a]Most patients will require 900-1500 mg/d to achieve pain control.
[b]There are multiple dosage formulations.
[c]Peak serum concentration of most short-acting oral morphine preparations occurs after 1 h; doses can be given as frequently as q2h without stacking/overlapping of doses.
[d]Initial dosing of short-acting oral morphine for opioid-naïve patients is 5-10 mg q4h PRN.
[e]Not appropriate for the initial management of acute pain.
[f]Initial dose of hydromorphone for opioid-naïve patients is 0.2-0.6 mg IV q2-3h PRN.
[g]Should only be used by those certified in conscious sedation and with appropriate monitoring/emergency equipment.

- Avoid IM injections. Subcutaneous opioids are equally efficacious and less painful than IM injections. Uptake can be erratic and unpredictable with both.
- Before prescribing pain medications, always consider comorbidities, allergies, drug interactions, and potential side effects.

- **Select alternative agents to meperidine and codeine** to limit potential side effects and drug interactions. At least 10% of the US population lacks the appropriate enzyme to convert codeine to the active compound morphine.

- One should always be aware of the "hidden" acetaminophen in combination products and not exceed the 4000 mg per day limit.[4] A lower dose for chronic administration should be considered (2000-3000 mg per day) in those with liver disease.[5]

- Consider obtaining a pain management consultation for other options in persistent, severe, uncontrolled pain.
    - Opioid-related deaths due to overdose have been increasing since the 1980s but have been rising even more sharply over the past 10 years.[6]
    - Patients receiving opioid prescriptions in addition to other sedating medications may be at a significant increased risk of oversedation, respiratory depression, and death.

- Neuromodulation, including low- and high-frequency nerve stimulation, may provide new treatment modalities in the coming years. In addition, as medical marijuana becomes legal in more states, providers will need to educate themselves on upcoming research regarding its role in pain management.

- Trust your instincts. If you think a patient is displaying aberrant drug-related behaviors, set boundaries and stick with them. Questions to ask:
    - Does the patient only ask for pain medications when you are in the room?
    - Do others observe different behaviors when you leave the room?
    - Is the patient "splitting" the staff, playing one against the other?
    - Is the patient talking or resting comfortably? This may be quite misleading in patients with chronic pain and should not be assumed to be a sign of deception in such patients.
    - Is the patient allergic to every pain medication except the one he/she is requesting?
    - Is the patient unwilling to accept any adjunctive nonopioid treatment?
    - Is the patient very sleepy or lethargic and still asking for more?

EQUIPOTENT ANALGESIC DOSES OF OPIOIDS

When transitioning to a PO pain regimen, the following steps can help calculate a starting dose. **Equipotent analgesic doses are approximate;** clinical conversions should be done carefully.

1. Calculate the total opioid dose used in the previous 24 hours.
2. Convert the total dose to an oral morphine equivalent using Table 13-2.
3. Convert from oral morphine equivalent to the new opioid.
4. Give 50% of the calculated daily dose to account for incomplete cross-tolerance between opioids. Conversion to or from methadone is not as straightforward (see Table 13-2).

TABLE 13-2	APPROXIMATE EQUIPOTENT OPIOID DOSES			
Drug	SQ/IV Dose (mg)	PO Dose (mg)	Duration (h)[a]	Half-Life (h)
Short half-life opioids				
Morphine	10	30	4	2-3.5
Hydrocodone	–	30	4	3-4
Oxycodone	–	20	4	3
Hydromorphone	1.5	7.5	4	2-3
Fentanyl	0.1	–	1-2	1.5-6
Long-acting opioids				
Methadone	–	1.7-6.7	4-48[b]	15-60[c]

[a] Duration of analgesic effect is for single-dose administration. To achieve steady state, it takes 5 half-lives; exert caution when starting long half-life opioids.
[b] Duration of analgesia for single-dose methadone is 4-8 h but increases to 12-24 h after achieving steady state. Total duration of action for methadone varies by person and chronicity of methadone use but is generally between 22 and 48 h.
[c] See the previous footnote. There is highly significant variability in the pharmacokinetic parameters of methadone.
When converting to methadone, use a starting dose of 10% of the 24 h IV morphine equivalent dose (24 h dose of IV morphine) × 0.10 = total daily methadone; divide by 2 for q12h, 3 for q8h dosing. Expect steady state in 5-7 d; dose adjust weekly.

5. Schedule the dosing frequency on the basis of the analgesic half-life (e.g., for morphine: q4h, MS Contin: q8-12h; oxycodone: q4h, OxyContin: q12h).

6. Divide the calculated 24-hour dosage by the number of doses to be given daily.

7. Add PRN doses of the new opioid (short-acting form) at 5% to 15% of the total daily dose for breakthrough pain.

References

1. Wong DL, Baker CM. Pain in children: comparison of assessment scales. *Pediatr Nurs* 1988;14:9-17.

2. Jaycox A, Carr DB, Payne R. New clinical practice guidelines for the management of pain in patients with cancer. *N Engl J Med* 1994;330:651-55.

3. World Health Organization. WHO's cancer pain ladder for adults. 2016. Available at: http://www.who.int/cancer/palliative/painladder/en/ (last accessed 11/3/17).

4. Food and Drug Administration. Notice to industry: final guidance for over-the-counter products that contain acetaminophen. Available at: https://www.fda.gov/Drugs/DrugSafety/ucm310469.htm (last accessed 11/3/17).

5. Chandok N, Wyatt KDS. Pain management in the cirrhotic patient: the clinic challenge. *Mayo Clin Proc* 2010;85:451-58.

6. Hedegaard M, Warner M, Minino AM. Drug overdose deaths in the United States, 1999-2015. *NCHS Data Brief.* 2017;273. Available at: https://www.cdc.gov/nchs/data/databriefs/db273.pdf (last accessed 11/3/17).

Fluids and Electrolytes

14

Thomas Hoyt and Steven Cheng

BASAL REQUIREMENTS

Water

- Basal water requirement may be calculated as follows:
  - What you were taught:

First 10 kg of body weight	4 mL/kg per hour	4×10
Second 10 kg of body weight	2 mL/kg per hour	2×10
Remaining weight > 20 kg	+1 mL/kg per hour	$1 \times n$
		= Hourly maintenance rate

  - What you should remember in adult medicine (if weight is >20 kg):
    - Body weight (kg) + 40 = hourly maintenance rate
    - That is, 60 kg (body weight) + 40 = 100 mL/kg per hour
- Increased insensible water loss occurs via fever, diaphoresis, and increased respiratory rate. Losses increase 100 to 150 mL/°C for each degree >37°C.

Electrolytes

- Sodium and chloride = 50 to 150 mmol per day (as NaCl). Most excreted in urine.
- Potassium = 20 to 60 mmol per day (as KCl). Most excreted in urine assuming normal glomerular filtration rate.

Carbohydrates

- Dextrose = 100 to 150 g per day
- IV dextrose minimizes protein catabolism and can help prevent ketoacidosis.

MAINTENANCE INTRAVENOUS FLUIDS

- **Maintaining the basal requirements noted above can be conveniently accomplished with 0.45% NaCl in 5% dextrose plus 20 mmol/L KCl (D5½NS + 20KCl).**

- Fluid losses are divided into urinary losses and all other losses.
  - Urinary losses in an average adult = 0.5 to 1 mL/kg per hour (e.g., for a 70 kg person ~40-60 mL/h or 1200 mL/d)
  - Other losses (via stool or insensible losses) ~800 mL/d
- Average-size adult = 2–3 L IV solution/day (D5½NS + 20KCl @ 100 mL/h).
- Consider the patient prior to resuscitation decision.
  - Hypovolemic patients will likely need more aggressive fluid resuscitation with normal saline.
  - Patients with heart or renal failure may require less fluid.
  - Patients with increased gastrointestinal (GI) or renal losses (e.g., diarrhea or diuretics) have more loss of H_2O, Na^+, and K^+. Closely monitor electrolytes in these patients.

ELECTROLYTE ABNORMALITIES

Hyponatremia

Etiology

- **Hypotonic hyponatremia**
  - Water intake is greater than water output.
  - Can be due to excessive water intake (primary polydipsia) or reduced water excretion due to the presence of antidiuretic hormone.
- **Isotonic hyponatremia** (pseudohyponatremia)
  - Decreased aqueous phase of plasma (e.g., hyperproteinemia, hyperlipidemia)
  - Na^+ per liter of plasma water is normal.
- **Hypertonic hyponatremia**
  - Increased extracellular solute concentration (e.g., hyperglycemia or IV mannitol)
  - Na^+ decreases by about 1.5 mmol/L for every 100 mg/dL glucose above normal.

Evaluation

- See Figure 14-1 for evaluation of hyponatremia.
- In the history and physical examination, be sure to check orthostatics, mucous membranes, skin turgor, jugular venous distension (JVD), and the presence of edema/ascites and perform a thorough neurologic examination.
- Minimum laboratory studies that are necessary include a plasma and urine osmolality and urine [Na^+].

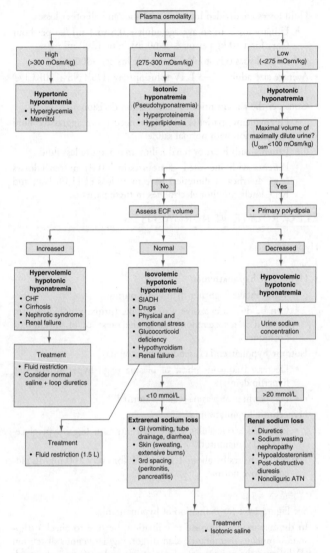

Figure 14-1. Evaluation of hyponatremia. ECF, extracellular fluid; CHF, congestive heart failure; SIADH, syndrome of inappropriate antidiuretic hormone; GI, gastrointestinal; ATN, acute tubular necrosis.

Treatment
- For mild or asymptomatic hyponatremia, consider just monitoring.
- For isovolemic/hypervolemic hypotonic hyponatremia, consider fluid restriction.
- In hypovolemic hypotonic, provide saline therapy.
- Correct slowly and steadily: In chronic hyponatremia, **overly rapid correction can lead to osmotic demyelination or central pontine myelinolysis.** (Note: This is bad. Avoid this.)
  - Chronic/asymptomatic: Correct 5 to 8 mmol/L over 24 hours.
  - Severe symptomatic (e.g., neurologic/central nervous symptom symptoms): often treated with hypertonic saline (requires very close monitoring, possibly in an intensive care unit). Correct 1 to 2 mmol/L for 3 to 4 hours (once stable, taper down, and don't exceed 10-12 mmol/L over 24 h).
- The quantity of Na^+ required to raise plasma Na^+ by a given amount is estimated as follows (TBW, total body weight):

$$Na^+ \text{ deficit (mmol)} = \text{desired change in } [Na^+] \times TBW$$

$$TBW = 0.6 \times \text{body weight (kg)}$$

- For a 70-kg patient, if the desired increase in $[Na^+]$ is 8 mmol, then 336 mmol of Na^+ would be required ($42 \times 8 = 336$). Can administer as 0.65 L 3% saline (336 mmol ÷ 513 mmol/L), or 2.2 L 0.9% (normal) saline (336 mmol ÷ 154 mmol/L).
- **No equation replaces the need for frequent Na^+ monitoring.**

Hypernatremia
Etiology
- Dehydration (more common)
  - **Water deficit**: decreased intake (e.g., patients with altered mentation, intubated patients), impaired thirst drive
  - **Water loss** via renal or extrarenal causes
- Rarely, from excess Na^+ intake (hypertonic saline or $NaHCO_3$)

Evaluation
- Perform a history and physical examination just like hyponatremia. Check mucous membranes, skin turgor, JVD, and the presence of edema or ascites and perform a thorough neurologic exam.
- Laboratory evaluation should include plasma/urine osmolality and urine $[Na^+]$. Refer to Figure 14-2.

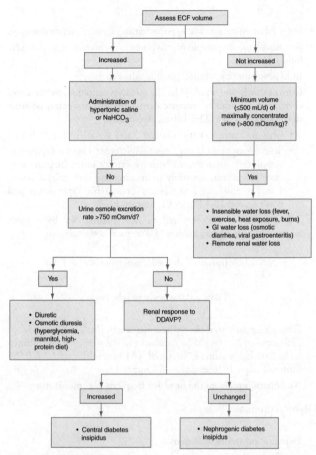

Figure 14-2. Evaluation of hypernatremia. ECF, extracellular fluid; GI, gastrointestinal.

Treatment

- Treat the underlying issues (e.g., hyperglycemia, diarrhea).
- In hypovolemic patients, restore extracellular fluid volume with isotonic saline.

$$\text{Free water deficit (L)} = (\text{plasma [Na}^+] - 140)/140 \times \text{TBW (L)}$$

$$\text{TBW} = 0.6 \times \text{body weight (kg)}$$

- As with hyponatremia, **correcting hypernatremia too rapidly is potentially dangerous.** The rate of plasma [Na⁺] correction should not exceed 0.5 mmol/L per hour (12 mmol/L in the first 24 h). This rate is even lower and slower in chronic asymptomatic hypernatremia: 5 to 8 mmol/L per day.
- Don't forget to take into account ongoing losses.
- Safest route is PO or nasogastric (NG) tube administration of water. Alternatively, ½NS, ¼NS, or D5W can be given intravenously.
- Reassess volume status and [Na⁺] every 8 to 12 hours.
- Diabetes insipidus (DI) management
    - Central DI is treated with intranasal Desmopressin (DDAVP).
    - Nephrogenic DI may be reversible by treating underlying disorder or removing offending agent (e.g., lithium).

Hypokalemia

- Defined as [K⁺] < 3.5 mmol/L.
- Clinical features vary, but myalgias and weakness are common.
- Severe hypokalemia leaves patients at increased risk of arrhythmias. In cardiac patients, the [K⁺] is generally maintained >4 mmol/L.

Etiology

- Decreased intake: very low K⁺ intake. This is rare because kidneys are able to conserve K⁺.
- Shifts: refeeding syndrome, insulin, β-adrenergic agonists, rising pH.
- Increased output: diarrhea, vomiting/NG suction, increased urine output (e.g., diuretics), hyperaldosteronism.
- Coexistent **hypomagnesemia** should be ruled out.

Evaluation

- When etiology not immediately apparent, renal K⁺ excretion and acid-base status can help identify the cause.
- The transtubular potassium gradient (TTKG) can help elucidate the source and is calculated by:

$$TTKG = (U_{[K^+]}/P_{[K^+]})/(U_{OSM}/P_{OSM})$$

    - TTKG <2 suggests a nonrenal source of K⁺ loss.
    - TTKG >4 suggests inappropriate renal K⁺ secretion.

- Acid-base status
  - Hypokalemia is generally associated with metabolic alkalosis.
  - Metabolic acidosis suggests lower GI losses, distal renal tubular acidosis, or diabetic ketoacidosis.

Treatment

- K^+ may be repleted orally or IV (note: the oral liquid tastes terrible). Generally, it is safer and more cost-effective to replace K^+ orally. The patient and your institution will like you better.
- Approximately 10 to 20 mmol of KCl is required to raise the serum level by 0.05 to 0.1 mmol/L. **Use caution in patients with renal insufficiency.**
- Use IV form in severe hypokalemia or if unable to tolerate PO.
  - Peripheral line: Do not administer >10 mmol/h.
  - Central line can tolerate > 20 mmol with ICU monitoring. >40 mmol/h only in life-threatening hypokalemia (ICU setting).
- Replete low magnesium levels as well.

Hyperkalemia

- Defined as $[K^+]$ > 5 mmol/L.
- The toxicity depends on acuity; the most serious complications involve cardiac toxicity. Gradual, chronic, modest hyperkalemia (5.0-5.6 mmol/L) is generally tolerated and often does not require aggressive treatment.
- If initial $[K^+]$ suspicious, get a stat whole blood level to confirm.
- **Always get an ECG** (refer to Chapter 16, ECG and Arrhythmias, for ECG interpretation).
  - Look for peaked T waves, prolonged PR or QRS intervals.
  - Consider telemetry.

Etiology

- Increased intake: huge K^+ intake
- Shifts: acidemia, β-blockers, cell lysis, diabetes, or digoxin (insulin deficiency or hyperglycemia)
- Decreased output: poor renal clearance (acute kidney injury, chronic kidney disease [CKD], or end-stage renal disease [ESRD]), low aldosterone state
- **Pseudohyperkalemia** (caused by K^+ movement out of cells): associated with venipuncture; may be seen with repeated fist clenching, prolonged tourniquet time, hemolysis, leukocytosis, or thrombocytosis

Evaluation

- Rule out pseudohyperkalemia (repeat serum electrolytes).
- Get a stat ECG and, if concerned for acidosis, an arterial blood gas.
- Assess the urine output and renal function.
- Examine the patient, paying particular attention to volume status.
- Review the medication list.

Treatment

- Stop all exogenous K⁺ and/or potentially offending drugs.
- Not all hyperkalemia requires immediate, aggressive treatment.
  - Particularly true of CKD/ESRD patients: often have mild hyperkalemia (5.0-5.6 mmol/L).
  - Unless clinical signs of significant hyperkalemia, acute management mentioned here is usually unnecessary.
- **Emergent treatment is required with severe hyperkalemia or hyperkalemia with ECG changes. Acute treatment includes the following:**
  - **Calcium gluconate** (10%, 10 mL [1 gm] IV over 2-3 min)
    - Can repeat after 5 to 10 minutes if no change in ECG.
    - Decreases cardiac membrane excitability.
    - Use with extreme caution in patients receiving digoxin.
  - **Insulin** (5-10 units IV)
    - Causes intracellular shift of K⁺, effect within 10 to 30 minutes (lasts several hours).
    - Coadminister glucose, 100 g IV (2 amps D50) to prevent hypoglycemia; remember to check blood glucose in 1 to 2 hours.
  - **NaHCO₃ 1 amp IV (50 mmol HCO₃⁻ in 50 mL)**
    - Causes intracellular K⁺ shift (effect lasts several hours).
    - Reserve for patients with severe hyperkalemia **AND** metabolic acidosis.
    - ESRD patients seldom respond and may not tolerate Na⁺ load.
  - **β2-Adrenergic agonists → intracellular shift of K⁺**
  - **Diuretics** (e.g., furosemide, 40-120 mg IV): enhance K⁺ excretion (if adequate renal function).

- **Cation exchange resins** (sodium polystyrene sulfonate, Kayexalate; patiromer) **enhance K⁺ excretion from the GI tract.**
  - Single doses are only mildly effective.
  - The FDA now recommends that Kayexalate NOT be given in sorbitol solution because of risk of intestinal necrosis.[1]
  - Kayexalate reconstituted in water may be given orally (15-30 g) or as an enema (50 g in 150 mL of tap water). May be beneficial to coadminister an alternative laxative (e.g., lactulose) when giving PO Kayexalate. Can repeat doses q4h.
  - Patiromer: initially dosed as 8.4 g daily (max dose: 25.2 g/d). Can increase dose qweekly in increments of 8.4 g.
- **Dialysis may be necessary for severe hyperkalemia if** aforementioned measures are ineffective and/or patients have renal failure.
- **Chronic treatment is aimed at the underlying condition.**
  - Dietary K⁺ should be restricted.
  - Metabolic acidosis should be corrected.
  - Medications causing hyperkalemia should be avoided.
  - Exogenous mineralocorticoids can help in certain patients.

Reference

1. Sanofi-Aventis. Kayexalate. 2009. Available at: https://www.accessdata.fda.gov/drugsatfda_docs/label/2009/011287s022lbl.pdf (last accessed 11/3/17).

Acid-Base Disorders

15

Stephanie Velloze and Timothy Yau

GENERAL PRINCIPLES

- Changes in acid-base balance occur as a result of changes in $[H^+]$ and $[HCO_3^-]$.
- **Acidemia** (pH <7.37) results from either decreased $[HCO_3^-]$ or increased PCO_2.
- **Alkalemia** (pH >7.43) results from either increased $[HCO_3^-]$ or decreased PCO_2.
- An arterial blood gas (ABG), electrolyte panel, and a serum $[HCO_3^-]$ are required to assess acid/base status.
- For a stepwise approach to evaluating an ABG, please see Figure 15-1. The steps are also outlined as follows:
    1. Examine the pH. Is the patient acidemic or alkalemic?
    2. Establish the primary disturbance.
        a. Examine the $[HCO_3^-]$ (must be obtained from basic metabolic panel). In primary metabolic disorders, it moves in the same direction as the pH (lower bicarb → more acid → lower pH).
        b. Examine the PCO_2. In primary respiratory disorders, it moves in the opposite direction as the pH.
        c. A combined disorder is present when (1) pH is normal but PCO_2 and $[HCO_3^-]$ are both abnormal or (2) PCO_2 and $[HCO_3^-]$ derange in opposite directions.
    3. Is there adequate respiratory or metabolic compensation? If there is not adequate compensation, there may be a combined disorder present. Compensation never fully corrects the pH to normal or "overshoots" in the opposite direction.
    4. If a metabolic acidosis is present:
        a. Calculate the anion gap (AG): $AG = [Na^+] - ([Cl^-] + [HCO_3^-])$. A normal AG is 10 to 12 and needs to be corrected for albumin ($AG_{correct} = AG + ([4-albumin] \times 2.5)$).
        b. If a normal gap is present, calculate the urine anion gap (UAG): $UAG = U_{[Na^+]} + U_{[K^+]} - U_{[Cl^-]}$. A negative UAG

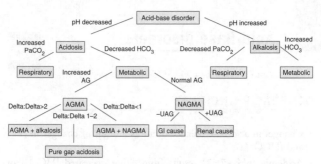

Figure 15-1. Algorithm for approaching acid-base problems. AG, anion gap; AGMA, anion gap metabolic acidosis; NAGMA, nonanion gap metabolic acidosis; GI, gastrointestinal.

suggests gastrointestinal [HCO_3^-] losses (ne-GUT-ive), whereas a positive UAG suggests renal losses such as a renal tubular acidosis.

5. If there is an increased AG, assess the delta gap:
   a. $\Delta AG = AG_{correct} - 12$.
   b. $\Delta[HCO_3] = 24 - [HCO_3]$.
   c. If they are approximately equivalent, there is a pure AG metabolic acidosis. This implies that the unmeasured anion leading to the increased gap is responsible for all of the acid production that is being buffered by the [HCO_3]. Lactic acidosis tends to be 1.6:1, whereas ketoacidosis tends to be closer to 1:1. If the ratio of $\Delta AG/\Delta[HCO_3]$ is >2, this indicates there is a lesser fall than one would expect in [HCO_3], so there is a coexisting metabolic alkalosis. If the ratio is <1, there is a greater fall in [HCO_3] than expected, indicating that there is both a gap and nongap acidosis.

METABOLIC ACIDOSIS

See Table 15-1 for etiology of AG metabolic acidosis and Table 15-2 for nonanion gap metabolic acidosis.

Treatment

- Treatment of the underlying condition should be the primary focus of all acid-base disturbances.
- Severe acidosis (pH <7.20) may require treatment with parenteral $NaHCO_3$.

TABLE 15-1	CAUSES OF ANION GAP METABOLIC ACIDOSIS
G	Glycols (ethylene, propylene either in isolation or as a vehicle for other medications)
O	Oxoproline (alternatively: other, for oxoproline and toluene)
L	L-Lactate
D	D-Lactate
M	Methanol
A	Aspirin
R	Renal failure
K	Ketones (diabetic, starvation, alcoholic)

- Options include bicarbonate (either in amp pushes or as a drip) or sodium acetate (converted to bicarbonate by the liver; cannot be bolused).
- One IV amp contains 50 mEq $NaHCO_3$.

TABLE 15-2	CAUSES OF NONANION GAP METABOLIC ACIDOSIS		
	GI Causes	Renal Causes	Others
	Diarrhea	Renal tubular acidosis	Ingestion of acids
	Urinary diversion	Early renal insufficiency	Expansion acidosis (rapid saline administration)
	Cholestyramine		Drug-induced hyperkalemia (K^+-sparing diuretics, trimethoprim, pentamidine, ACE inhibitors, nonsteroidal anti-inflammatory drugs, cyclosporine), carbonic anhydrase inhibitors
	Ingestion of CaCl or MgCl		
	Small bowel and pancreatic fistulas		

GI, gastrointestinal.

- Mild nonanion gap metabolic acidosis can be supplemented with oral bicarbonate tablets. One 650 mg tablet contains 7.8 mEq of $NaHCO_3$.
- Overaggressive correction should be avoided to prevent overshoot alkalosis.
- Adverse effects of parenteral $NaHCO_3$ include volume overload, hypercapnia, hypernatremia, hypokalemia, and hypocalcemia. Monitor electrolytes frequently.

METABOLIC ALKALOSIS

Etiology

- Metabolic alkalosis may be caused by $[HCO_3^-]$ gain, H^+ loss, or volume contraction.
- Vomiting and diuretic use are the two most common causes.
- See Table 15-3 for etiologies of metabolic alkalosis.

TABLE 15-3 CAUSES OF METABOLIC ALKALOSIS	
Cl⁻ Responsive (Urine Cl⁻ <10 mmol/L)	Cl⁻ Unresponsive (Urine Cl⁻ >10 mmol/L)
Gastrointestinal	**Normotensive**
Vomiting, NG suction	K^+ or Mg^{2+} depletion
Villous adenoma	Bartter syndrome
Congenital chloridorrhea	Hypercalcemia
Cystic fibrosis	Refeeding syndrome
Renal	**Hypertensive**
Diuretics	Hyperreninemic hyperaldosteronism
Posthypercapnic state	Primary hyperaldosteronism
Nonreabsorbable anions (penicillin)	**Adrenal enzyme defects**
Exogenous alkali ($NaHCO_3^-$ massive transfusion, antacids, acetate, citrate)	Hypercortisolism
Contraction alkalosis	Mineralocorticoid excess-like states (licorice ingestion, Liddle syndrome)

NG, nasogastric.

Treatment

- Correct hypokalemia and hypomagnesemia.
- **Chloride-responsive metabolic alkaloses** should be treated with isotonic normal saline.
- Chloride-unresponsive metabolic alkaloses do not improve with saline administration. K^+-sparing diuretics (e.g., amiloride, triamterene, spironolactone) are effective for mineralocorticoid excess states.
- In patients with normal renal function, alkalosis from excessive alkali administration will resolve quickly once the $[HCO_3^-]$ load is withdrawn.
- Acetazolamide may be useful if alkalosis persists despite the aforementioned interventions or if saline administration is limited by volume overload.
- In severe alkalosis, or in conditions where renal function is impaired, dialysis against a low bicarbonate bath can be performed. Alternatively, intravenous infusion of hydrochloric acid can be administered only via central access in an ICU setting.

RESPIRATORY ACIDOSIS

Etiology

- Increased PCO_2 is almost always the result of alveolar hypoventilation.
- In **acute respiratory acidosis**, the pH $\downarrow 0.08$ for every 10 mm Hg $\uparrow PCO_2$ above 40 mm Hg.
- In **chronic respiratory acidosis**, the pH $\downarrow 0.03$ for every 10 mm Hg $\uparrow PCO_2$ above 40 mm Hg.
- Renal compensation takes several days to develop fully.
- See Table 15-4 for causes of respiratory acidosis.

Treatment

- Potentially contributing drugs should be stopped or counteracted (e.g., naloxone, flumazenil).
- Ventilatory assistance may be required (continuous positive airway pressure, bilevel positive airway pressure, or invasive mechanical ventilation).
- Avoid $NaHCO_3$ administration, as this can worsen hypercapnia ($[HCO_3^-]$ combines with H^+ in the tissues to form $CO_2 + H_2O$ via carbonic anhydrase).

TABLE 15-4	CAUSES OF RESPIRATORY ACIDOSIS

Central respiratory depression (drugs, sleep apnea, obesity, CNS disease)

Airway obstruction (foreign body, laryngospasm, severe bronchospasm)

Neuromuscular abnormalities (polio, kyphoscoliosis, myasthenia, muscular dystrophy, C3-5 spinal injury)

Parenchymal lung disease (COPD, pneumothorax, pneumonia, pulmonary edema, interstitial lung disease)

CNS, central nervous system; COPD, chronic obstructive pulmonary disease.

RESPIRATORY ALKALOSIS

Etiology

- It is important to remember that tachypnea/hyperventilation does not necessarily imply a simple respiratory alkalosis. If you have any uncertainty, obtain an ABG.
- See Table 15-5 for causes of respiratory alkalosis.

Treatment

Psychogenic hyperventilation may be treated by rebreathing from a paper bag.

TABLE 15-5	CAUSES OF RESPIRATORY ALKALOSIS

Central nervous system causes (e.g., CVA, ICH, psychogenic)

Hypermetabolic (hyperthyroidism, pregnancy, sepsis/fever, anxiety, pain)

Environmental (hyperthermia)

Drugs (aspirin, progesterone)

Liver failure

Hypoxemia (pneumonia, PE, congenital heart disease, altitude compensation)

Iatrogenic (mechanical ventilation)

CVA, cerebrovascular accident; ICH, intracerebral hemorrhage; PE, pulmonary embolism.

ECG and Arrhythmias

16

Samuel Reinhardt and Justin Sadhu

TACHYCARDIA

- Tachyarrhythmias are defined by a ventricular rate of greater than 100 bpm and are broadly categorized as either a wide-complex tachycardia (WCT) (QRS duration ≥120 ms) or a narrow-complex tachycardia (NCT) (QRS <120 ms).

- **In the unstable patient with a tachyarrhythmia (e.g., hypotension, altered mental status, ischemic chest discomfort, acute heart failure, or other signs of shock), immediately ask for help, initiate ACLS protocols, and place defibrillator pads to prepare for electrical cardioversion.**

- In an otherwise stable patient, some time and thought can lead to a satisfying diagnosis!

Narrow-Complex Tachycardias

- NCTs, characterized by a QRS duration <120 ms, are almost **always supraventricular in origin.** When dealing with NCTs, it is useful to first assess **whether the rhythm is regular or irregular** (Figure 16-1).

- If the tachyarrhythmia is **regular,** examine a standard 12-lead ECG for p-waves. The rhythm can then be further categorized by assessing whether the p-wave is closer to the R-wave that precedes it (**short R-P tachycardia**) or the R-wave that follows it (**long R-P tachycardia**).

- In the case of **long R-P tachycardia,** consider the diagnoses of (1) sinus tachycardia, (2) ectopic atrial tachycardia, or (3) atrial flutter.

- For **short R-P tachycardia,** consider (1) atrioventricular (AV)-nodal reentrant tachycardia (AVNRT) and (2) atrioventricular reentry tachycardia (AVRT).

- If the tachyarrhythmia is **irregular,** the diagnosis is almost always (1) atrial fibrillation, (2) atrial flutter (with variable block), or (3) multifocal atrial tachycardia (MAT).

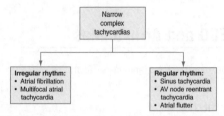

Figure 16-1. Common narrow-complex tachycardias.

Sinus Tachycardia
Key Features

- Characterized by **usual P-wave morphology** (positive deflection in leads II, III, and aVF) and a rate generally between 100 and 160 bpm. Sinus tachycardia is almost never faster than (220 − patient age) bpm; if an NCT is faster than this, suspect another cause of tachycardia.
- Remember, sinus tachycardia is almost **always secondary to another process.**
- If telemetry data are available at the onset of the arrhythmia, a graph of heart rate (HR) over time will typically show a gradual increase to the fast rate with sinus tachycardia, whereas other NCTs will show an abrupt change in rate, indicating the change in rhythm from sinus.

Management

- In patients with underlying causes for sinus tachycardia such as hypovolemia, pulmonary emboli, or myocardial infarction (MI), an elevated HR may be the patient's only means for maintaining cardiac output (cardiac output = HR × stroke volume), and thus treatment of sinus tachycardia in these patients with negative chronotropic agents (β-blockers, calcium channel blockers) is ill-advised.
- Other potential causes include infection, anemia, anxiety, exertion, thyroid disease, administration or withdrawal from certain drugs or other substances, autonomic neuropathy (especially of diabetes), and inflammation.
- A thorough workup for underlying causes should be pursued before sinus tachycardia is treated with medications that slow down the HR.
- In the patient without heart failure, intravenous fluids aid in the management of many conditions that cause sinus tachycardia and may be a useful starting point in management.

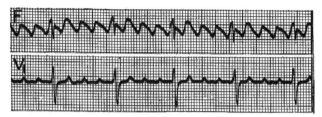

Figure 16-2. Atrial flutter.

Atrial Flutter
Key Features

- Atrial flutter results from large reentrant circuits within the atria. There are several types of atrial flutter. This rhythm should be suspected when the **atrial rate is around 300 bpm** (1 big box between the flutter waves) (Figure 16-2).

- Characterized by flutter waves in a regular, undulating (wavelike), sawtooth pattern at a rate of 280 to 350 bpm. Flutter waves are best seen in leads II, III, aVF, and V1.

- Because the AV node cannot usually conduct impulses at a rate greater than 180 bpm, the ventricular rate corresponding to atrial flutter is usually slower and frequently around 150 bpm (2:1 AV conduction).

- One frequent misdiagnosis occurs when the ECG is read as "sinus tachycardia with first-degree heart block" with a ventricular rate of around 150 bpm. In this case, look closely for any flutter waves that may be buried within the QRS interval. Here, comparison to an old ECG in sinus rhythm can be helpful to identify any subtle changes in the QRS complex arising from the superimposed flutter wave.

Management

- Management of atrial flutter is very similar to that of atrial fibrillation (see Atrial Fibrillation section); consideration must be given to rate control, rhythm control, and anticoagulation.

- **Rate control is often harder to achieve in atrial flutter than in atrial fibrillation, so anticoagulation followed by direct current cardioversion may be the best strategy for some patients.** (Transesophageal echocardiogram is recommended to exclude atrial thrombus if the duration is greater than 48 h.)

Atrioventricular Nodal Reentrant Tachycardia and Atrioventricular Reentry Tachycardia

Key Features

- AVNRT and AVRT arise from related but pathophysiologically distinct mechanisms.

- **AVNRT occurs in the presence of conduction tissues of differential speeds and refractoriness within the AV node, often described as a "fast pathway" and a "slow pathway."** The tachycardia is **often triggered by a premature atrial contraction** that travels down (antegrade) the slow pathway (**manifested as a prolonged PR interval**) and then retrograde back up the fast pathway (short RP interval).

- AVRT can occur in the presence of a muscular bridge/accessory conduction pathway between the atria and ventricles that is independent of the AV node.

- AVNRT typically occurs at a rate of around 180 to 200 bpm but can be slower.

- **AVRT tends to run slightly faster (200 bpm) than AVNRT, but there is significant overlap in the possible rates of the two rhythms.**

- Strongly suspect one of these rhythms when a tachycardia is regular at rates >170 bpm.

Management

- As always, in the hemodynamically unstable patient, call for help, initiate ACLS if necessary, and prepare for electrical cardioversion!

- **In the hemodynamically stable patient, attempt to make a diagnosis by "breaking the rhythm." This is done by temporarily blocking conduction through the AV node to either terminate the rhythm (if reentrant) or else unmask the underlying atrial activity. The latter can be useful with fast atrial flutter or sinus tachycardia when the underlying atrial rhythm is not clear.**

- This can be done by first asking the nurse to set up a 12-lead ECG and run a rhythm strip.

- Initially, ask the patient to perform **vagal maneuvers** (i.e., Valsalva).

- If this does not work, listen for carotid bruits and, if there are none and low suspicion for carotid disease, attempt unilateral carotid massage.

- Never attempt bilateral simultaneous **carotid massage**, given the risk of cerebral hypoperfusion!

- If neither of these breaks the rhythm, ask for help and have a nurse bring vials of adenosine to the bedside.

- **Adenosine** will temporarily block conduction through the AV node, terminating AVRT or AVNRT.
  - To administer adenosine, have a nurse place a y-stopcock onto a standard IV. Prepare the patient by telling him/her that he/she may experience an unpleasant sensation upon administration.
  - Always have the defibrillator close by if cardioversion or pacing is required.
  - Have the nurse push adenosine 6 mg IV followed immediately by a saline flush, as adenosine will otherwise be rapidly metabolized in the arm prior to reaching the heart.
  - If this does not produce a satisfactory result, repeat the same maneuver with 12 mg of adenosine.
  - If the adenosine has successfully blocked AV-nodal conduction but the rhythm is not in fact AVRT or AVNRT, QRS complexes will be suppressed, and only atrial activity will appear on the rhythm strip. This may reveal flutter waves or a nonsinus p-wave (as in ectopic atrial tachycardia).

Ectopic Atrial Tachycardia
Key Features

- A sinus p-wave should be positive in leads II, III, and aVF and negative or biphasic in lead V1, with a PR interval of 120 to 200 ms.
- If a long-RP NCT has a P-wave morphology unlike that of a sinus P-wave, the rhythm is likely ectopic atrial tachycardia.
- It is useful to distinguish ectopic atrial tachycardia from sinus tachycardia, as the search for underlying causes will differ.

Management
Management of ectopic atrial tachycardia is geared toward slowing conduction through the AV node, usually with β-blockers or calcium channel blockers (see Atrial Fibrillation section).

Atrial Fibrillation
Key Features

- The mechanisms underlying atrial fibrillation are still being elucidated, but the end result is disorganized atrial activity at a rapid rate, usually in the range of 300 to 600 bpm.
- Atrial fibrillation in the absence of heart block demonstrates an **irregularly irregular R-R interval** and no regular P-waves, although you may see coarse atrial activity or fibrillatory waves (Figure 16-3).
- **For new onset atrial fibrillation and atrial flutter, consider workup for underlying causes.**

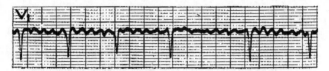

Figure 16-3. Atrial fibrillation.

- A convenient mnemonic for common causes of atrial flutter or fibrillation is PIRATES: Pulmonary disease (e.g., chronic obstructive pulmonary disease [COPD] or pulmonary embolism), Ischemia (i.e., acute MI), Rheumatic or valvular heart disease, Anemia, Thyrotoxicosis, Ethanol/Electrolytes, Sepsis.
- Because the AV node cannot usually conduct at rates >180 bpm, if the ventricular response is at a higher rate, suspect the presence of an accessory pathway with ventricular preexcitation.

Management
- In the hemodynamically stable patient, rate-control is typically the first priority; consider whether a rhythm-control strategy is also warranted.
- **Rate control can typically be achieved with AV-nodal blocking agents: nondihydropyridine calcium channel blockers (e.g., diltiazem), β-blockers such as metoprolol, or digoxin** (digoxin may be better tolerated in patients with low blood pressure or heart failure).
  - **Diltiazem** can be given as an IV push, with a typical initial dose of 10 to 15 mg, followed by a continuous infusion (usual starting dose of 5 mg/h, titrated as tolerated for goal HR <100 bpm and SBP >100 mm Hg).
  - **Metoprolol** is usually given in increments of 5 mg IV, with up to three consecutive doses at 5-minute intervals, followed by a PO regimen, such as 12.5 mg PO q6h. This can then be titrated until HR control is achieved.
  - **Digoxin**, while also a negative chronotrope, is not an antihypertensive, making it useful for slowing the HR in patients with lower blood pressures. Digoxin can be proarrhythmic, and caution should be exercised when using this medication in patients with low body weight, impaired renal function, or electrolyte abnormalities. Digoxin may be given in increments of 0.25 mg IV q6-8h or as oral doses (please see a more complete text for dosing instructions). Keep in mind that digoxin will take longer to exert its effect than diltiazem or metoprolol.
  - Ask for help prior to using other agents such as amiodarone, as these confer a risk of cardioversion.

- **Electrolyte repletion** is essential in atrial fibrillation. Specifically, the potassium should be >4.0 mEq/dL and magnesium >2.0 mEq/dL.

- **Anticoagulation** should also be considered, depending on the patient's risk of stroke, regardless of whether sinus rhythm can be restored. The commonly accepted thromboembolic risk-stratification tool is the CHA_2DS_2VASc score.[1]

- For new atrial fibrillation of unknown period or period greater than 48 hours in a patient not on therapeutic anticoagulation, care must be taken to avoid cardioversion with pharmacologic or electrical means because of the risk of thromboembolism.

Multifocal Atrial Tachycardia
Key Features

- MAT is an irregularly irregular rhythm that is the result of multiple distinct foci of pacemaker activity within the atria.

- It is identified by the presence of **three or more distinct P-waves** that reliably give rise to QRS complexes.

- Each P-wave should have a unique morphology and PR interval because of its distinct location in the atria in relation to the surface electrocardiographic leads and the AV node.

- MAT usually occurs in the presence of significant underlying pulmonary disease, most commonly COPD.

Management

Management is similar to that for atrial fibrillation using rate control with a β-blocker or calcium channel blocker and electrolyte repletion. However, there is no role for digoxin, and anticoagulation is not needed. Treat the underlying condition.

Wide-Complex Tachycardias

- WCTs are characterized by a QRS duration of ≥120 ms. At the beginning of your internship, you should always ask for help before attempting to manage patients with WCT!

- In the hemodynamically unstable patient with WCT, time to defibrillation is the strongest predictor of survival and favorable outcome. As always with an unstable patient, call for help, initiate ACLS protocol, and place defibrillator pads to prepare for electrical cardioversion/defibrillation if necessary.

- In the stable patient, a WCT can be the result of a supraventricular rhythm (including sinus tachycardia) with bundle branch block, a supraventricular rhythm with aberrant conduction, or ventricular tachycardia (VT).

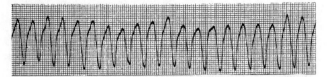

Figure 16-4. Ventricular tachycardia.

- Key features on history, labs, and the ECG can help make the diagnosis.
- **In a patient with structural heart disease or history of MI, a WCT is almost always VT, assuming that the patient does not have underlying bundle branch block** (Figure 16-4).
- The presence of capture or fusion beats on ECG clinches a diagnosis of VT as well.
- There have been numerous proposed algorithms to aid in the diagnosis of WCT as supraventricular tachycardia versus VT, the most well-known of which is the Brugada Criteria, found elsewhere.[2]
- Management of stable WCT depends on the diagnosis.
- In the case of VT, options include electrical cardioversion or attempted pharmacologic cardioversion.
- In the case of SVT, management is per the "Narrow-Complex Tachycardias" section.
- In either case, the patient is at high risk for decompensation, and you should call for help before initiating treatment!

Nonsustained Ventricular Tachycardia
Often as an intern, you will be called for "beats of nonsustained ventricular tachycardia (NSVT)" or "a run of NSVT." NSVT is defined as **fewer than 30 seconds** of consecutive wide-complex beats (>120 ms) that are ventricular in origin with HR >100 bpm.

- These usually occur in patients with heart failure or toxin ingestion. If the patient is hemodynamically stable, nothing needs to be done on an emergent basis, but **assess for electrolyte abnormalities (especially K^+, Mg^{2+}), ischemia, and medications that may prolong the QT interval.**
- As always, if the patient demonstrates hemodynamic instability or altered mental status during the episodes, ask for help, as the patient likely requires treatment.
- In most patients with NSVT, **adding/increasing a β-blocker as tolerated is the best initial management**, and antiarrhythmic medications are not necessary.

- NSVT alone is rarely an indication for placement of an implantable cardioverter-defibrillator.

Sustained Ventricular Tachycardia
Key Features

- As opposed to NSVT, sustained VT lasts more than 30 seconds or is associated with hemodynamic instability.
- VT can be monomorphic (single QRS morphology) or polymorphic (multiple QRS morphologies).

Management

- If you cannot easily determine that the WCT is SVT with aberrancy, it should be treated as VT, and you should call for help immediately!
- Sustained VT in an unstable patient should be treated immediately with DC cardioversion by ACLS protocol.
- In patients with hemodynamically stable VT, pharmacologic treatment may be attempted using amiodarone, lidocaine, or less commonly procainamide. This should only be done in the presence of your senior resident and/or a cardiology fellow.
- As VT may degenerate into ventricular fibrillation (VF) and death, defibrillation pads should be placed on the chest of any patient with sustained VT.

Ventricular Fibrillation and Torsades De Pointes

- **Close this book and call a code!** These rhythms should prompt immediate initiation of ACLS and rapid defibrillation.
- VF is characterized by completely chaotic, rapid, highly variable amplitude electrical activity originating in the ventricles. There are no regular QRS complexes, as both electrical and mechanical activities are disorganized, resulting in no effective cardiac output. **These patients require emergent defibrillation.**
- Torsades de Pointes (TdP) is a rapid, polymorphic VT with QRS complexes that oscillate in amplitude and morphology, which appears as a twisting axis of depolarization.
- TdP usually occurs in the setting of a prolonged QT interval (from electrolyte abnormalities or offending medications) and a premature ventricular complex.
- If TdP does not terminate spontaneously, unstable patients require electrical cardioversion.
- In the case of TdP, IV magnesium sulfate 1 to 2 g IV may aid restoration of normal sinus rhythm if the patient is hemodynamically stable. Offending medications that prolong the QT interval should be discontinued.

BRADYARRHYTHMIAS AND DISORDERS OF CONDUCTION

Sinus Bradycardia

- Sinus bradycardia is defined as sinus rhythm (P-waves with positive deflection in II, III, and aVF) with a rate of less than 60 bpm.
- **Sinus bradycardia is most often caused by increased vagal tone; medications, including antiarrhythmic agents; ischemia; and primary sinoatrial node dysfunction, aka "sick sinus syndrome"** (may be seen with long-standing hypertension, diabetes, or increased age).
- Sinus bradycardia is common in sleeping patients.
- Sinus bradycardia should be **treated only if there are attributable symptoms or hypotension.** That is to say, if you are called for sinus bradycardia, and the patient is asymptomatic with an acceptable blood pressure, the patient likely requires no urgent treatment.
- Look for offending agents that can cause bradycardia, such as β-blockers, calcium channel blockers, digoxin, or other medications. Discontinue these unless otherwise indicated.
- Acute treatment can consist of the anticholinergic agent atropine and/or placement of pacing pads with transcutaneous pacing.
- Atropine can be given in increments of 0.5 mg IV, every 3 to 5 minutes to a max dose of 3 mg, until the HR is satisfactory.
- Atropine has a half-life of 2 hours, so after resolution with atropine, care must be taken to ensure the bradycardia does not return.
- Infusions such as dopamine or isoproterenol can be considered as pharmacologic means to restore and maintain the HR. Call for help prior to initiating these treatments.
- Transcutaneous pacing should be employed if necessary but is exceedingly uncomfortable for the patient. Transvenous pacing should be considered in the symptomatically bradycardic patient, with the help of an upper level resident or cardiology fellow.

First-Degree Atrioventricular Block
Key Features

- The PR interval is greater than 200 ms, but all P-waves result in a QRS complex (Figure 16-5).
- First-degree block can be caused by increased vagal tone, electrolyte abnormalities, conduction system degeneration, and drugs (calcium channel blockers, β-blockers, and antiarrhythmic agents are common causes). Ischemia can in specific instances prolong the PR interval.

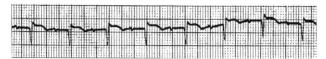

Figure 16-5. First-degree atrioventricular block.

Management

- First-degree block rarely requires treatment. If severe, consideration can be given to discontinuation of offending drugs.
- First-degree block with progressive PR interval prolongation can occur in patients with aortic root abscess. Consider this diagnosis in a patient with aortic valve endocarditis and first-degree block, as it requires surgical intervention.

Second-Degree Atrioventricular Block

In second-degree block, not all P-waves result in a QRS complex.

Mobitz Type I Block (Wenckebach)
Key Features

- In second-degree block, not all P-waves result in a QRS complex.
- Mobitz I is identified when the **PR interval progressively increases** between PQRS complexes, until a p-wave is not conducted to the ventricle and does not result in a QRS complex (Figure 16-6).
- Mobitz I usually occurs as a result of slowed conduction within the AV node.
- The QRS complexes should not change in morphology.
- Etiologies are the same as for first-degree block.
- Mobitz type I block is usually asymptomatic.

Management

- Given that it is asymptomatic and **does not usually progress to worsening heart block, this type of block requires no urgent treatment.**
- If symptomatic bradycardia ensues, treatment is the same as that for sinus bradycardia.

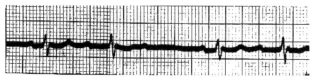

Figure 16-6. Mobitz type I (Wenckebach), second-degree atrioventricular block.

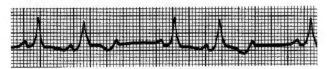

Figure 16-7. Mobitz type II, second-degree atrioventricular block.

Mobitz Type II Block

Key Features

- In second-degree block, not all P-waves result in a QRS complex.
- Mobitz type II block is diagnosed when **the PR interval is fixed, but one or more P-waves fail to conduct, i.e., do not result in a QRS complex** (Figure 16-7).
- Mobitz II usually occurs as a result of slowed conduction just below the AV node.
- Blocked conduction may occur in a fixed ratio (two, three, or four conducted P-waves for one nonconducted P-wave).
- Causes are similar to Mobitz type I block.

Management

- **Because Mobitz type II block is at high risk for degenerating into complete AV block, these patients must be closely monitored.**
- Treatment usually involves placement of external pacer pads, regardless of symptoms, so that they are ready in case the patient becomes hemodynamically unstable and requires external pacing. Most patients with this diagnosis should be in an ICU or step-down unit for close monitoring.

Third-Degree (Complete) Atrioventricular Block

Key Features

- **No P-waves are conducted; complete AV dissociation occurs** (Figure 16-8).

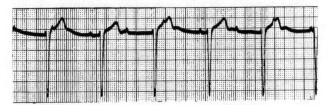

Figure 16-8. Complete heart block.

- QRS complexes that arise do so as the result of intrinsic pacemakers within or below the level of the AV node.
- "Escape" rhythms usually occur in the acute setting and obviate the development of asystole. If a narrow QRS occurs, the rhythm originates from the AV node's intrinsic pacemaker and is referred to as "junctional." If a wide QRS occurs, the rhythm originates from somewhere within the ventricles and is termed "idioventricular."

Management

- **Third-degree block carries a high risk of degeneration to asystole.**
- Therefore, regardless of symptoms, patients need to be monitored in an ICU and have external pacer pads placed in case external pacing becomes necessary. Once in the ICU, a plan for short-term **transcutaneous and/or transvenous pacer can be discussed.** Eventual permanent pacemaker placement is the definitive therapy.

Escape Rhythms

- Stimulation of the His-Purkinje system and the ensuing QRS complex is driven by the fastest active intrinsic pacemaker within the heart. Usually, this is the sinus node.
- In the event of sinus node failure, the AV node's pacemaker may assume pacemaking responsibilities for the heart, resulting in a junctional rhythm. **Junctional rhythm** can be recognized when a narrow-complex QRS (or a QRS similar to the one caused by sinus rhythm) arises without any detectable atrial activity (P-waves) and has a regular rhythm. The rate is usually between 40 and 60 bpm.
- In the event of failure of both the junctional and sinus pacemakers, pacemakers within the ventricle may resume pacemaking responsibilities. If this occurs, the rhythm is termed "**idioventricular rhythm.**" Because the pacemakers are located within the ventricle, conduction does not necessarily occur through the His-Purkinje system, and the QRS complex is wide. The rate is typically around 40 bpm. Thus, idioventricular rhythm can be identified by a wide, regular, and slow rhythm that occurs independently of atrial activity.
- **Treatment is the same as for patients with third-degree heart block.** Your resident or fellow should be called, and plans for increasing the HR using drugs such as dopamine or dobutamine or temporary pacing should be considered.

MYOCARDIAL ISCHEMIA

General Principles

- Remember to keep the clinical picture in mind when interpreting ECGs. In the symptomatic patient with chest pain or other anginal equivalent, very subtle ECG changes could represent significant ischemia. Likewise, in the asymptomatic patient, consider whether you would have ordered an ECG in the first place. As always, if you are unsure, ask for help!
- **When confronted with a patient with suspected ischemia, it is always useful to obtain an old ECG for comparison!** If the patient has baseline abnormalities on the old ECG, changes from that baseline could represent a pathologic process.

ECG Findings

ST Segment and T-Waves

- Myocardial ischemia is characterized by symmetric T-wave inversion, flat or downsloping ST depression, or both.
- ST elevation MI (STEMI), representing severe ischemia, will present with ECG changes as shown in Figure 16-9, depending on when in the pathologic process the ECG is taken.
- The distribution of leads in which ECG changes representing ischemia are observed can often help localize the region of myocardium that is ischemic (Table 16-1).
- If changes are observed in leads **I and aVL, ischemia likely involves the high lateral wall**; the culprit vessel is typically a proximal diagonal artery or the circumflex artery.
- If changes are observed in leads **II, III, and aVF, ischemia likely involves the inferior wall**; the culprit lesion is likely in the distal circumflex artery or right coronary artery.
- Changes in leads **V1-V2 represent the septal region** of the heart; consider a left main or proximal left anterior descending (LAD) lesion.
- Changes in **V3-V5 represent a continuum of myocardium extending from the anterior LV to lateral LV**; consider mid- to distal LAD and proximal to mid-circumflex lesions.
- In a symptomatic patient, **a new LBBB could represent severe ischemia**, and you should immediately call for help!
- Keep in mind that in patients with known LBBB, there will be some anteroseptal ST segment elevation and lateral ST segment depression. Likewise, in RBBB, there will be some anteroseptal ST depression.

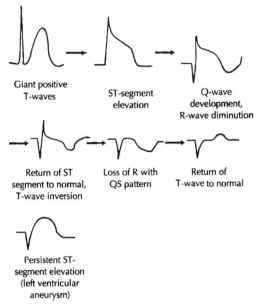

Figure 16-9. ST- and T-wave changes in ST elevation myocardial infarction.

- Similarly, patients with LVH or on digoxin (Figure 16-10) will often have lateral ST segment depression, and interpretation of those changes as ischemic or nonischemic must be made taking into account all clinical factors (e.g., symptoms) and laboratory values (e.g., cardiac enzymes).

R-Waves

- The utility of precordial R-waves in interpreting ECGs is often underappreciated.
- Examining leads V1-V6 sequentially, the R-wave should be larger than the S-wave by lead V3 and larger in each subsequent lead than the previous. If this pattern is not present, the patient is said to have poor R-wave progression.
- The differential for **poor R-wave progression** includes obesity, incorrect lead placement, and pulmonary disease; however, in the setting of a patient who is suspected of having myocardial ischemia, poor R-wave progression could represent the equivalent of a q-wave. The interpretation of an ECG with poor R-wave progression should read "cannot

TABLE 16-1	ECG LOCALIZATION OF MYOCARDIAL INFARCTION (MI)	
Area of MI	**ECG Abnormality**	**Artery Involved**
Septal	ST elevation and Q-waves in V1-V2	Proximal left anterior descending (LAD), septal perforators
Anteroseptal	ST elevation and Q-waves in V1-V4	LAD
Anterior	ST elevation and Q-waves in V3-V4	LAD
Anterolateral	ST elevation and Q-waves in I, aVL, V3-V6	Mid-LAD or circumflex
Extensive anterior	ST elevation and Q-waves in I, aVL, V1-V6	Proximal LAD
Lateral	ST elevation and Q-waves in I, aVL, V6	Circumflex
High lateral	ST elevation and Q-waves in I, aVL	Circumflex
Inferior	ST elevation and Q-waves in II, III, aVF	Right coronary artery (RCA)
Posterior	Tall R and ST depression V1-V2	RCA or circumflex
Right ventricular	ST elevation V4R	Proximal RCA

rule out anterior infarct, age indeterminate." As always, interpret the ECG in the setting of all clinical and laboratory information at hand.

- The true posterior region of the myocardium is poorly represented on the standard 12-lead ECG. The presence of a tall R-wave in lead V1 with ST depression should alert the clinician to a possible posterior STEMI. Call for help if you note this ECG finding in the symptomatic patient!

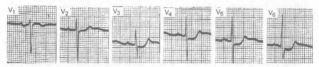

Figure 16-10. Digitalis effect.

Q-Waves

- Pathologic Q-waves are longer than 40 ms in duration and larger than one-third the total QRS amplitude or one-fourth the R-wave amplitude.

- Q-waves usually represent a region of infarcted myocardium and should typically be observed in 2 or more contiguous leads. Non-pathologic Q-waves can be seen in leads III and aVR and in isolation do not necessarily indicate infarction.

- However, as always in the symptomatic patient, have a lower threshold for recognizing a change as acute, and pay close attention to newly found Q-waves.

Management

Management of acute myocardial ischemia should usually involve your resident. Having the patient chew nonenteric-coated aspirin 325 mg PO is always a good starting point. See Chapter 12, Top 10 Workups, for further information on evaluation of acute chest pain.

Conditions Mimicking ST-Elevation Myocardial Infarction

- Certain other conditions beyond MI will also cause ST elevations on the ECG.

- **Pericarditis is associated with diffuse ST elevations** (Figure 16-11). Certain clues, however, can point away from the diagnosis of STEMI. Clinically, the patient may have the classic pericarditis presentation, with chest pain and shortness of breath that is relieved with leaning forward or with NSAIDs. The patient may also have historical features (e.g., recent upper respiratory infection) that predispose to pericarditis. On ECG, the ST elevations will often not follow a single arterial distribution. Classically, the ECG will also show depression of the PR segment. Meanwhile, lead aVR typically shows PR elevation and ST depression.

- **Takotsubo cardiomyopathy (or "stress cardiomyopathy") can also cause diffuse ST elevations.** Takotsubo cardiomyopathy is an increasingly recognized condition that occurs during episodes

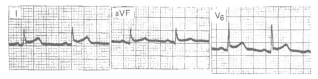

Figure 16-11. Pericarditis.

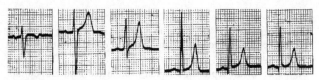

Figure 16-12. Hyperkalemia.

of great emotional or physiologic stress; patients present with symptoms similar to those of acute MI and with positive cardiac biomarkers. ECG may show ST elevations and anterior precordial T-wave inversions with segmental myocardial wall motion abnormalities on imaging. Takotsubo cardiomyopathy occurs in the absence of epicardial coronary artery occlusion but is a diagnosis of exclusion and may require cardiac catheterization to exclude significant CAD.

- **Ventricular aneurysms** may occur as a late sequela of a STEMI. Clues to this diagnosis include the presence of ST elevations in a patient with prior STEMI but without new symptoms and with normal cardiac biomarkers. The diagnosis is confirmed with ventricular imaging such as echocardiography.
- **Severe hyperkalemia**, usually with levels greater than 5.5 mg/dL, can present with **sharply peaked T-waves**, imitating the changes found during the hyperacute phase of a STEMI (Figure 16-12). As hyperkalemia worsens, the QRS will widen. Strongly suspect hyperkalemia in a patient with known renal disease or on high doses of spironolactone, ACE inhibitors, or angiotensin receptor blockers. In the setting of hyperkalemia, ECG changes should trigger immediate medical treatment (see Chapter 14, Fluids and Electrolytes, for more details).

References

1. Lip GY, Nieuwlaat R, Pisters R, et al. Refining clinical risk stratification for predicting stroke and thromboembolism in atrial fibrillation using a novel risk factor-based approach: The Euro Heart Survey on atrial fibrillation. *Chest* 2010;137:263-72.
2. Brugada P, Brugada J, Mont L, et al. A new approach to the differential diagnosis of a regular tachycardia with a wide QRS complex. *Circulation* 1991;83:1649-59.

Radiology

17

Anup Shetty and Sanjeev Bhalla

INTRODUCTION

Interpreting basic radiographs will likely be an important component of your training. This chapter will walk you through what radiologists look at in chest radiographs and abdominal plain films. This chapter also discusses preparation for specific radiology testing, adverse reactions, and different imaging modalities.

PLAIN FILMS

Chest Radiograph

- The chest radiograph (CXR) is by far the most common imaging study you will order and need to interpret.
- The importance of a systematic approach to the CXR cannot be overstated. Mistakes happen when shortcuts are taken. **Be sure to check the name and date on the image and compare with old images whenever possible.** See Figure 17-1 for CXR examples.

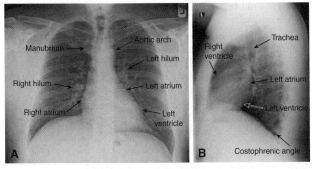

Figure 17-1. A. Posteroanterior chest radiograph. **B.** Lateral chest radiograph.

Technique

- Are the windowing and exposure correct?
  - Underexposure or narrow windows can cause you to see things that aren't there, whereas overexposure or wide windows can cause pathology to disappear.
  - You should be able to faintly see the intervertebral disk spaces through the cardiac silhouette.
- Is the patient properly positioned?
  - The spinous processes and trachea should be midline.
  - The clavicular heads should be equidistant from the spinous processes.
  - Rotated films distort the appearance of the cardiac silhouette and hila.
- Is the frontal image posterior-anterior (PA) or anterior-posterior (AP)?
  - AP images are often obtained in emergent situations or when the patient cannot stand.
  - A two-view (PA and lateral) examination is optimal if the patient can tolerate it.
  - A normal cardiac silhouette will appear magnified on an AP exam because of its proximity to the X-ray source.
- Was the image taken at full inspiration?

  Small lung volumes can produce vascular crowding, apparent mediastinal widening, and atelectasis.

Lines and Tubes

- If the patient is intubated, check the position of the endotracheal tube (should be a minimum of 2 cm above the carina with 3 to 5 cm optimal).
- Central venous catheters should follow expected venous courses and should generally terminate at the superior cavoatrial junction, approximately two vertebral body levels below the carina along the right aspect of the mediastinum. The end of the catheter should travel along the long axis of the superior vena cava (vertically).
- Nasogastric and enteric feeding tubes may be partially visualized. Ensure they do not coil in the esophagus or extend outward into the lung because of endobronchial placement.

Airway

- The trachea should be midline and not deviated.
- The trachea will deviate away from the side of a pneumothorax if there is tension physiology. In cases of volume loss such as lobar collapse, it will deviate toward the affected side.

Bones

Systematically evaluate the sternum, ribs, clavicles, spine, and shoulders for fractures, osteolytic or osteoblastic lesions, and arthritic changes.

Diaphragm

- The sides of the diaphragm should be equal and slightly rounded. The right side may be slightly higher. Elevation of one side may suggest subpulmonic effusion, paralysis, loss of lung volume on that side, diaphragmatic eventration, or diaphragmatic injury in the setting of trauma.
- Blunting of the costophrenic angles suggests small pleural effusions, evaluated more sensitively on the lateral view (approximately 50 mL vs. 300 mL of fluid).
- Flattened hemidiaphragms are indicative of hyperexpansion, often seen in emphysema.
- Check for free air under the diaphragm on an upright radiograph, which can be seen with bowel perforation. If you think you've detected free intraperitoneal air, let your resident know right away! Something is clearly very wrong.

Soft Tissues

Examine the soft tissues for symmetry, subcutaneous air, edema, and breast tissue.

Heart and Mediastinum

- Maximal heart width greater than half of the chest width suggests cardiomegaly or pericardial effusion.
- The aortic knob should be distinct.
- Mediastinal widening may indicate thoracic aortic dissection or aneurysm, lymphadenopathy, or mass. In obese patients, it may be related to mediastinal fat deposition.
- Mediastinal and tracheal deviation can be seen with a tension pneumothorax. The trachea will deviate away from the side of the pneumothorax if tension physiology is present.
- Use lateral images to confirm findings on frontal images and look for retrocardiac pathology, such as lower lobe pneumonias or hiatal hernias.

Hilar Structures

- The left hilum is usually 2 to 3 cm higher than the right. Both hila are generally of equal size.
- Enlarged hila suggest lymphadenopathy or pulmonary artery enlargement. Use the lateral image to help differentiate.

Lung Markings

- Look for normal lung markings all the way out to the chest wall to rule out pneumothorax. If lung markings are not seen to the periphery, look for a thin white visceral pleural line. Be sure not to miss this! If you think you've detected a pneumothorax, let your resident know right away!

- Normal lung markings taper as they travel out to the periphery and are smaller in the upper lungs. Lung markings in the upper lung zones that are as large as or larger than those in the lower lung (so-called cephalization) suggest pulmonary edema.

- Kerley B lines (small linear densities perpendicular to the pleural surface often best seen in the lung bases) are seen in heart failure.

- Hyperlucent lungs with increased retrosternal clear space on the lateral image are seen in emphysema.

- Examine the lungs for areas of consolidation and nodules.

- Obscuration of all or part of the heart border (silhouette sign) implies that a lesion is contiguous with or abuts the heart border and likely lies within the right middle lobe or lingula.

- A small pleural effusion is suggested by blunting of the costophrenic angle, best seen on the lateral image. Larger effusions obscure the shadow of the diaphragm and produce an upward-curving shadow along the chest wall. A straight horizontal air-fluid level indicates a concurrent pneumothorax (hydropneumothorax).

- Lateral decubitus films can be done to ensure that the effusion is free flowing and large enough to attempt thoracentesis (usually >1 cm on lateral film). The side of the effusion should be down.

Abdominal Films

- Ordered quite frequently, abdominal radiographs (KUB [kidneys, ureters, and urinary bladder] or obstructive series) are usually a first-line screening study, and subsequent studies may be needed to clarify or identify pathology.

- An obstructive series consists of a frontal image and left lateral decubitus or upright image and should be ordered when evaluating for perforation or small bowel obstruction. Again, a systematic approach is key. See Figure 17-2 for abdominal film examples.

Bones

- Examine the bones first or else you'll forget. And really, who wants to forget "dem bones?"

- Begin with the spine, and then the ribs, pelvis, and upper femurs. Look for arthritis, fractures, and osteolytic or osteoblastic lesions.

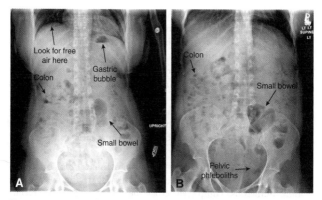

Figure 17-2. A. Upright abdominal film. **B.** Supine abdominal radiograph.

Lines and Tubes

- Nasogastric/orogastric tubes should terminate in the left upper quadrant, with the proximal-most side port past the gastroesophageal junction.
- Enteric feeding tubes should course past the stomach into the right abdomen and then cross back over the midline to the left (following the course of the duodenum) to terminate in the jejunum.

Soft Tissues

- Systematically study the soft tissues looking for evidence of masses or calcifications. Calcifications can be seen over the gallbladder, pancreas, renal shadows, or course of the ureters; in the right lower quadrant (appendicolith); or overlying the uterus (fibroids). Phleboliths (vascular calcifications) are commonly seen in the pelvis and usually have a lucent center.
- Be sure to carefully look for free air under the diaphragm (upright film) or next to the liver edge (left lateral decubitus film). A supine radiograph is typically insufficient to assess for free air. Free air is indicative of bowel perforation. If you see this, let your resident know immediately! Essentially never a good finding, unless there's a really good explanation.

Gastrointestinal Structures

- Look for the gastric bubble. A large air-distended stomach suggests some form of obstruction or dysfunction. Burp.

- Observe the bowel gas pattern. A small amount of air is generally seen in the colon, while the small bowel is frequently devoid of air. Fecal material is often visible in the colon although large amounts may be seen in constipation.
- The colon may become distended (colon diameter >6 cm or cecum >9 cm) in colonic obstruction or ileus. Unless the distension is severe, the haustral markings are maintained. Large bowel markings are differentiated from small bowel markings by wider spacing and incomplete crossing of the lumen. When the ileocecal valve is incompetent, large bowel obstruction may also cause gaseous distension of the small bowel.
- Distension of the small bowel (>3 cm in diameter) may be seen in mechanical obstruction or ileus. Small bowel striations are much more numerous, completely cross the lumen, and may become effaced with dilatation.
- With mechanical obstruction, there is distension proximal to the obstruction and decompression of air distally. The appearance of ileus is much less distinct. There is discontinuous air in the small and usually large bowel. The degree of distension is also less remarkable.
- Air-fluid levels unfortunately do not always distinguish mechanical obstruction from ileus, as they may be seen in both conditions.

OTHER IMAGING MODALITIES

There is a myriad of imaging modalities these days, including CT, MRI, and ultrasound. See Table 17-1 for indications for some advanced imaging. This section will also discuss general preparation for other imaging, adverse reactions, and information on specific modalities.

Preparation for Procedures

- Perform plain radiographs prior to contrast studies. Perform iodinated contrast studies prior to barium studies. Barium can cause metallic streak artifact on CT, which obscures findings to the point that it may preclude the exam until the barium is cleared from the bowel.
- Consult your radiology department if you have questions about what study to order or to confirm preparation for procedures. Some preparations are institution specific (see Table 17-2).
- Studies requiring no preparation include chest and abdominal radiographs, cervical spine series, transthoracic echocardiogram, and those listed in Table 17-2.

| TABLE 17-1 | INDICATIONS FOR RADIOLOGICAL STUDIES |

Test	Indication
CT chest without contrast	Pulmonary parenchymal disease, pleural effusions, pneumothorax, pulmonary nodules, interstitial lung disease
CT chest with contrast	Vascular disease such as pulmonary embolism and aortic dissection, lung cancer staging, mediastinal disease, left ventricular assist device–related complications
CT abdomen/pelvis without contrast	Nephrolithiasis, retroperitoneal hematoma, bowel obstruction
CT abdomen/pelvis with contrast	Virtually everything else in the abdomen and pelvis
CT abdomen/pelvis with and without contrast	Liver/pancreatic/renal lesion characterization, bowel ischemia, gastrointestinal bleeding, active bleeding elsewhere
CT head without contrast	Stroke, altered mental status, trauma
Abdominal ultrasound	Abnormal liver function tests, cholelithiasis/cholecystitis, cirrhosis, ascites
Renal ultrasound	Acute kidney injury, hydronephrosis, renal stones, renal masses
Pelvic ultrasound	Abnormal uterine bleeding, ovarian pathology, uterine fibroids

- Studies requiring the patient to be NPO include CT scans with contrast, abdominal ultrasound, gastrointestinal (GI) studies, cholescintigraphy (HIDA [hepatobiliary iminodiaceticacid]) scan, positron emission tomography scan, and those listed in Table 17-2.
- Remember to restart the diet postprocedure or if the procedure is canceled.

Adverse Reactions

Contrast Reactions

- Everyone feels a sense of warmth or flushing and many patients experience nausea and/or vomiting during contrast administration—these are not allergies. It's sort of like the first week of internship.

TABLE 17-2   PREPARATION FOR RADIOLOGY TESTS

Procedure	Preparation
CT	
Chest/extremity/head	Usually none if noncontrast. If intravenous contrast is to be administered, the patient should be NPO for 4-6 h.
Abdominal/pelvic	No intravenous (IV) contrast needed if looking for renal stone or retroperitoneal bleed. Other types of studies usually require IV contrast if possible and may require oral, depending on the patient and the indication. Discuss special protocol needs (liver, pancreas, renal protocol) and need for oral contrast with the radiologist.
MRI	If IV contrast is to be administered, the patient should be NPO for 4-6 h; sometimes oral contrast material will be given.
Ultrasound	
Abdominal	NPO starting 6 h prior to procedure.
Pelvic	4 glasses of water 1 h prior; no voiding 1 h prior to exam.
Gastrointestinal (GI) studies	
Barium swallow (used to evaluate pharynx and esophagus typically for dysphagia workup)	NPO 6 h prior to procedure.
Modified barium swallow (used to evaluate for possible aspiration during feeding)	NPO if concern for aspiration.
Upper GI (used to evaluate the esophagus, stomach, and proximal small intestine; typically used to look for ulcers)	NPO starting midnight the day of procedure.

Small bowel follow-through (contrast is followed through the small intestine; typically used to evaluate for areas of stricture or large mucosal abnormalities)

NPO starting midnight the day of the procedure.

Barium enema (used to evaluate the colon for mucosal lesions such as polyps and strictures)

NPO after midnight; bowel prep varies by indication. Consult the radiology department.

Cholescintigraphy (HIDA scan)

NPO starting midnight the day of procedure.

PET scan

NPO starting midnight the day of procedure. In diabetic patients, glucose must be under reasonable control (200 mg/dL).

Genitourinary studies

Cystogram

No dietary restriction, full bladder.

Interventional studies

If the patient is having a procedure that will require sedation (almost all procedures other than tube or line change), the patient should be NPO 4-6 h before the exam.

Endoscopic studies

Upper endoscopy/endoscopic retrograde cholangiopancreatography

NPO starting 6 h prior to procedure.

Colonoscopy

Clear liquids 1 d prior to procedure; 1 gallon of polyethylene glycol 3350 and electrolytes (e.g., GoLYTELY) 1 cup per 15 min until done on the night prior to procedure (consider NG tube if not able to complete); NPO after midnight.

Flexible sigmoidoscopy

Clear liquids starting with dinner the night before; NPO after midnight. Magnesium citrate at 8:00 p.m., 1 glass of water every 2 h until 10 p.m., then 3 bisacodyl tablets at 10:00 p.m., and 1 bisacodyl suppository at 6 a.m.

HIDA, hepatobiliary iminodiacetic acid; PET, positron emission tomography.

- For known contrast sensitivity (e.g., hives, rash), consider prednisone, 50 mg PO q6h × 3 doses prior to the exam. The last dose should be administered 1 hour prior to the administration of contrast. Diphenhydramine, 50 mg PO, can also be added, 1 hour prior to contrast. Specific protocols vary by institution, so be sure to double-check.

- Only nonionic contrast is used for CT (check your institution for confirmation); however, if your patient has had a major event with previous contrast administration (e.g., shock or airway compromise), discuss this with the radiologist prior to ordering a test. Patients who have had life-threatening reactions in the past should not receive intravenous contrast again, even with premedication. Allergic reactions generally do not occur with PO contrast.

- The contrast used in MR examinations is a gadolinium preparation, not iodinated contrast. There is cross-reactivity in some patients; therefore, those with severe contrast reaction to nonionic intravenous CT contrast should receive premedication for gadolinium contrast as well. See aforementioned premedication regimen. Those with only mild sensitivity generally do not require premedication.

- There is a relationship between gadolinium administration and nephrogenic systemic sclerosis in the setting of impaired renal function. Patients with creatinine clearance <30 mL/min or acute kidney injury and/or those on dialysis are at higher risk. Consult with your radiologist about preparatory regimens, reduction in the gadolinium load, or performing the study without contrast.

Contrast Nephropathy

- Contrast nephropathy is a potential complication of any procedure involving iodinated IV contrast (e.g., radiological studies, angiograms).

- Controversy exists as to whether contrast-induced nephropathy is a discrete process or coincident in patients who would otherwise develop acute kidney injury.

- Risk factors include the presence of renal insufficiency, diabetes, reduced intravascular volume, and large amounts of infused contrast.

- Strategies for prevention include the following:
  - IV hydration: 1 mg/kg per hour of 0.45 or 0.9 NS for 6 to 12 hours before and 6 to 12 hours after the procedure. A sodium bicarbonate solution, 3 ampules of $NaHCO_3$ (150 mEq total) in 1 L D5W, can also be used. This much $NaHCO_3$ should not be put in saline because of the high sodium load.

- *N*-acetylcysteine 600 mg bid × 2 doses before the procedure and 2 doses after the procedure may also be added **but is of uncertain benefit in most patients.**
- The risks and benefits of IV contrast should be weighed cautiously in patients with a Cr >2.0 and those with acute kidney injury.

Specific Imaging Modalities

Gastrointestinal Radiology

- GI studies can be uncomfortable and require patient cooperation and mobility. If your patient is paralyzed, demented, angry, or delirious, the study will likely be suboptimal or may not be performable or diagnostic. If you are demented, angry, or delirious, it largely doesn't matter.
- General rules for the barium versus Hypaque (i.e., diatrizoate) dilemma (call the radiologist if you have specific questions):
  - Barium is bad in pleural or peritoneal spaces, so avoid this if perforation, obstruction, or a fistula is suspected. Do not use if the patient is likely to need a laparotomy or CT soon.
  - Hypaque is bad in lungs, so avoid in cases of possible aspiration.

Cardiac Studies

- In general, no smoking 2 hours prior to test.
- Remove nicotine patches the morning of the test.
- Small sips of water with medication are fine; however, depending on the type of exam certain cardiac medications (i.e., β-blockers) may need to be held. Consult with the radiology department. For specific recommendations, refer to Table 17-3.

MRI

- Absolute contraindications are (most) pacemakers, implantable cardiac defibrillators, cochlear implants, any metal in the globe, and ferromagnetic intracranial aneurysm clips. Patients with so-called MRI-compatible pacemakers still require careful monitoring during the exam and close coordination with radiology when ordering the study.
- Relative contraindications are recent operations (less than a few weeks) and recent vascular stenting. Prosthetic hip joints or metal implants are not generally contraindicated, but their artifact may obscure any adjacent lesions. If you have questions, consult MRIsafety.com (last accessed 1/2/18) or call the radiologist.

TABLE 17-3	PREPARATION FOR CARDIAC TESTS
Test	**Preparation**
Coronary angiogram	NPO after midnight.
Stress echo, dobutamine stress echo, or exercise stress test	NPO after midnight. Hold AM doses of calcium channel blockers and β-blockers.
Nuclear stress test (walking)	NPO after midnight. Hold AM doses of calcium channel blockers and β-blockers.
Adenosine or dipyridamole nuclear stress test (nonwalking)	For diabetics on insulin only, half the normal insulin dose and eat a light meal 3 h prior to procedure (no fats or dairy products). Avoid any xanthine-containing products (e.g., chocolate, caffeine) and theophylline or dipyridamole for 24 h prior to procedure.

- These examinations can be relatively long. The patient must be able to lie still and cooperate—consider mild sedation (e.g., lorazepam) if necessary. The tube is quite small, and patients may get claustrophobic.

Ultrasound

- Abdominal ultrasounds can be used to evaluate the gallbladder, liver, bile ducts, and kidneys. The pancreas is typically not well visualized, so consider CT instead.
- Ultrasound can also locate pockets of fluid to guide paracentesis or thoracentesis.
- It is important the patient be made NPO because bowel gas can obstruct visualization.

Anticoagulation Management

18

Jennifer Riney, Jane Portell, and Ed Casabar

ANTICOAGULATION

- Before initiating anticoagulant therapy, ensure that the patient has no history of active peptic ulcers, recent stroke or bleeding, or recent surgery.
- All patients should have a digital rectal examination to document stool occult blood status.
- As required by The Joint Commission, for the laboratory tests that should be performed at baseline and during maintenance therapy to reduce patient harm, please see Table 18-1.

UNFRACTIONATED HEPARIN WEIGHT-BASED DOSING

- Typical initial bolus (round to the nearest 100 units)
  - Acute myocardial infarction (MI): 60 units/kg, maximum 4000 units

TABLE 18-1	LAB TESTS TO OBTAIN PRIOR TO AND DURING ANTICOAGULATION
Anticoagulant	**Required Lab Tests**
Warfarin	Baseline: CBC, PT/INR, PTT in previous 48 h
	Maintenance: CBC and PT/INR q72h
Enoxaparin	Baseline: CBC, PT/INR, PTT, serum creatinine in previous 48 h
	Maintenance: CBC and serum creatinine q72h
Heparin infusion	Baseline: CBC, PT/INR, PTT in previous 48 h
	Maintenance: PTT q6h until therapeutic ×2, then q24h, CBC q72h

CBC, complete blood count; PT, prothrombin time; INR, international normalized ratio; PTT, partial thromboplastin time.

TABLE 18-2	WEIGHT-BASED DOSING OF UNFRACTIONATED HEPARIN	

PTT (s)	Bolus	Infusion Rate
<40	3000 units[a]	↑ by 3 units/kg per hour
40-50	2000 units[b]	↑ by 2 units/kg per hour
51-59	None	↑ by 1 units/kg per hour
60-94	None	No change
95-104	None	↓ by 1 units/kg per hour
105-114	None	Hold 30 min, ↓ by 2 units/kg per hour
≥114	None	Hold 60 min, ↓ by 3 units/kg per hour

PTT, partial thromboplastin time; DVT, deep venous thrombosis; PE, pulmonary embolism.
[a]Acute DVT/PE: higher bolus (e.g., 80 units/kg) is recommended (typical max dose is 6000 units).
[b]Acute DVT/PE: a higher bolus (e.g., 40 units/kg) can be used (typical max dose is 6000 units).

- Acute deep venous thrombosis (DVT)/pulmonary embolism (PE): 80 units/kg, maximum 6000 units
- Non-DVT/PE or acute MI: 60 units/kg, maximum of 6000 units
- High risk of bleeding: consider smaller bolus
- Typical initial IV infusion rate
  - Acute MI: 12 units/kg per hour, maximum 1000 units/h
  - Acute DVT/PE: 18 units/kg per hour. If BMI >40, consider 14 units/kg per hour
  - Non-DVT/PE or acute MI: 14 units/kg per hour
  - High risk of bleeding: consider 12 units/kg per hour
- Check activated partial thromboplastin time (aPTT) 6 hours after initial bolus and 6 hours after each rate change. If two consecutive aPTTs are therapeutic, the aPTT should be monitored each morning.
- Complete blood count should be monitored every 72 hours while on IV heparin.
- Dosage adjustments based on aPTT are shown in Table 18-2.

LOW-MOLECULAR-WEIGHT HEPARIN DOSING

- **Enoxaparin:** 1 mg/kg subcutaneously (SC) q12h (unstable angina, non-ST-elevation MI [NSTEMI], or venous thromboembolism [VTE]). For DVT/PE, 1.5 mg/kg q24h is an alternative. If creatinine clearance (CrCl) <30 mL/min, use 1 mg/kg SC q24h. At BJH, for lung transplant patients with DVT/PE, 0.8 mg/kg SC q12h is used.

- **Dalteparin**: 120 units/kg SC q12h (unstable angina or NSTEMI) or 200 units/kg SC q12h (VTE).
- **Fondaparinux** (synthetic selective factor Xa inhibitor): 7.5 mg SC q24h (DVT/PE); use 5 mg SC q24h if weight <50 kg, and 10 mg SC q24h if weight >100 kg.
- For all acute coronary syndrome (ACS) patients, round doses down to nearest 10 mg. For all others, round to the nearest 10 mg.
- Individual hospitals are likely to have established protocols for low-molecular-weight heparin (LMWH) use in ACS. The enoxaparin ACS protocol at Barnes-Jewish Hospital is presented in Table 18-3.

TABLE 18-3	ENOXAPARIN ACS (ACUTE CORONARY SYNDROME) PROTOCOL FROM BARNES-JEWISH HOSPITAL	
Indication	Estimated CrCl (mL/min)	Enoxaparin Dose (Note: Round Down to Nearest 10 mg for ACS)
NSTEMI	>30	1 mg/kg SC q12h
	10-30	1 mg/kg SC q24h
STEMI	>30	Age <75 y • 30 mg IV bolus × 1 • With 1 mg/kg SC q12h × 2. Max 100 mg/dose for the first 2 doses • Then 1 mg/kg SC q12h Age ≥75 y • No IV bolus • 0.75 mg/kg SC q12h × 2 doses. Max of 75 mg/dose for the first 2 doses • Then 0.75 mg/kg SC q12h
	10-30	Age <75 y • 30 mg IV bolus × 1 • With 1 mg/kg SC × 1 • Then 1 mg/kg SC q24h Age ≥75 y • No IV bolus • 1 mg/kg SC q24h

CrCl, creatinine clearance; NSTEMI, non-ST-elevation myocardial infarction; STEMI, ST-elevation myocardial infarction.

- Dosages need to be adjusted in patients with renal failure; unfractionated heparin is recommended for patients with a CrCl <10 mL/min or on hemodialysis. Anti-Xa monitoring may be considered in the following situations: pregnancy, renal insufficiency (CrCl <40 mL/min), and morbid obesity (BMI >40). Draw peak anti-factor Xa (anti-Xa) level 4 hours after the 4th dose.
- Risk of bleeding is increased in patients with anti-Xa levels above 0.8 units/mL.
- Dosing in patients with a BMI >40 is uncertain. Monitoring anti-Xa levels is recommended in these patients.
- There is currently no validated nomogram for adjusting LMWH dosing on the basis of anti-Xa levels in adults.

DABIGATRAN

- Capsules should not be opened, crushed, chewed, or given per tube.
- Avoid coadministration with P-glycoprotein (P-gp) inducers (e.g., carbamazepine, rifampin, trazodone, St. John's Wort).
- For acute treatment of DVT/PE, start only after the patient has received 5 to 10 days of parenteral anticoagulation.
- Atrial fibrillation or DVT/PE: 150 mg PO bid. Dose adjustment required in the presence of renal dysfunction and/or drug interactions.

RIVAROXABAN

- Avoid use in moderate to severe hepatic dysfunction (Child-Pugh B or C) or any hepatic disease associated with coagulopathy.
- Avoid coadministration with P-gp and CYP3A4 inhibitors (e.g., ketoconazole, itraconazole, clarithromycin, boosted lopinavir, ritonavir, boosted indinavir, or conivaptan) or inducers (e.g., carbamazepine, phenytoin, rifampin, St. John's Wort).
- Atrial fibrillation: 20 mg PO q24h with evening meal (renally adjusted if CrCl <50 mL/min).
- DVT/PE: 15 mg PO bid with food for 3 weeks, followed by 20 mg PO q24h with food. Avoid use if CrCl <30 mL/min).

APIXABAN

- Atrial fibrillation: 5 mg PO bid.
- VTE treatment: 10 mg PO bid for 7 days, then 5 mg PO bid for 6 months. For extended prophylaxis after 6 months: 2.5 mg PO bid.

- Avoid coadministration with dual strong CYP3A4 and P-gp inhibitors (e.g., ketoconazole, clarithromycin, itraconazole, boosted lopinavir, ritonavir, boosted indinavir, or conivaptan).
- Dose adjustment required for age, body weight, renal function, presence of CYP3A4 or P-gp inhibitors, or cirrhosis.

WARFARIN DOSING

- **Warfarin dosing must be individualized!**
- The onset of action of warfarin is 24 to 72 hours, but full effect is not achieved until 5 to 7 days.
- Numerous common drugs increase the effect of warfarin including amiodarone, azole antifungals, fluoroquinolones, macrolides, metronidazole, trimethoprim-sulfamethoxazole, NSAIDs, acetaminophen, and proton-pump inhibitors.
- Drugs that decrease the effect of warfarin include carbamazepine, phenobarbital, phenytoin, rifampin, and ritonavir.
- Initial and subsequent dosing of warfarin may be guided by WarfarinDosing.org (last accessed 1/2/2018), which has been widely used and scrutinized.

Atrial Fibrillation/Atrial Flutter

- Generally, the goal international normalized ratio (INR) is 2 to 3.
- For cardioversion, if rhythm has been present >48 hours, anticoagulate for 3 weeks prior to procedure (or perform transesophageal echocardiogram prior to cardioversion) and 4 weeks afterward.
- For patients with chronic or paroxysmal atrial fibrillation (rate or rhythm control), calculate $CHADS_2$ score: 1 point each for Congestive heart failure, Hypertension, Age >75 years, Diabetes (DM); 2 points for prior ischemic Stroke or transient ischemic attack. See Table 18-4 for treatment recommendations based on $CHADS_2$ score.

Venous Thromboembolism Prophylaxis
See Table 18-5 for VTE prophylaxis recommendations.

Venous Thromboembolism Treatment
See Table 18-6 for VTE prophylaxis recommendations.

Heart Valve Replacement
See Table 18-7 for heart valve replacement treatment recommendations.

TABLE 18-4	TREATMENT OPTIONS FOR STROKE PREVENTION BASED ON CHADS$_2$ SCORE.[a]		

CHADS$_2$ Score[b]	Stroke Rate[c]	95% CI	Recommended Therapy
0	1.9	1.2-3.0	**Preferred**: no therapy **Alternative**: aspirin 81-325 mg qday
1[d]	2.8	2.0-3.8	**Preferred:**
2	4.0	3.1-5.1	• Warfarin with INR goal 2-3, or
3	5.9	4.6-7.3	• Dabigatran[e]
4	8.5	6.3-11.1	• CrCl >30 mL/min: 150 mg bid
5	12.5	8.2-17.5	• CrCl 15-30 mL/min: 75 mg bid
6	18.2	10.5-27.4	• Rivaroxaban[e] • CrCl >50 mL/min: 20 mg qday with evening meal • CrCl 15-50 mL/min: 15 mg qday with evening meal • CrCl <15 or HD: not recommended • Apixaban[e] • Most patients: 5 mg bid • If ≥2 of the following: 2.5 mg bid • Age ≥80 y • Body weight ≤60 kg • SCr ≥1.5 mg/dL • CrCl <25 mL/min: avoid use • Child-Pugh Class C or D: avoid use **Alternative:** • Alternative for patients at high risk for bleeding: aspirin 81-325 mg • Alternative for patients that are not anticoagulation candidates for reasons other than bleeding risk: aspirin 81 mg daily + clopidogrel 75 mg daily

CrCl, creatinine clearance; HD, hemodialysis.
[a]Therapy is lifelong unless contraindications exist.
[b]See text for the description of the CHADS$_2$ score.
[c]Expressed as rate per 100 person-years.
[d]For patients with CHADS$_2$ score of 1, additional risk factors for stroke (female gender, vascular disease, or age 65-74 y) should be considered.
[e]See text regarding coadministration with other agents.

TABLE 18-5	VENOUS THROMBOEMBOLISM (VTE) OPTIONS	
Risk Category	Recommended VTE Prophylaxis	
No VTE risk factors	Ambulation ± elastic stockings	
With VTE risk factors, nonambulatory	• **< 50 kg**: UFH 5000 units SC bid • **50-100 kg**: UFH 5000 units SC bid or tid[a] • **>100 kg and BMI >40**: UFH 7500 units SC tid[a]	Not considered first-line therapy at BJH: • Enoxaparin 40 mg SC q24h[b] • Fondaparinux 2.5 mg SC q24h[c]
Trauma patients	• **<50 kg**: UFH 5000 units SC bid • **50-100 kg**: enoxaparin 30 mg SC bid (if CrCl <30: UFH 5000 units SC tid) • **>100 kg and BMI >40**: Enoxaparin 40 mg SC bid (if CrCl <30: UFH 7500 units SC tid)	–
Orthopedic patients	• **Enoxaparin**: 30 mg SC bid[b] • **Warfarin**: INR 1.8-2.2 (2-2.5 with additional VTE risk factors) • **<50 kg**: UFH 5000 units SC bid	• Rivaroxaban: See text for prescribing details • ASA 325 mg PO bid

Neurosurgery patients	• **Enoxaparin**:
	  • **BMI ≥40**: 40 mg SC daily
	  • **BMI <40**: 30 mg SC daily
	  • **CrCl <30 mL/min**: order heparin SC
	• **Heparin**:
	  • **<50 kg**: 2500 units SC bid
	  • **51-79 kg**: 5000 units SC bid
	  • **≥80 kg**: 5000 units SQ tid[a]
		Fondaparinux (only if history of assay-confirmed HIT): >50 kg and CrCl >50: 2.5 mg SC daily[c]

UFH, unfractionated heparin; BMI, body mass index; BJH, Barnes-Jewish Hospital; CrCl, creatinine clearance (mL/min); INR, international normalized ratio; HIT, heparin-induced thrombocytopenia.

[a]Standard heparin tid times: 0600, 1300, and 2100.
[b]If >100 kg and BMI >40: 40 mg SC q12h. If CrCl 10-30 mL/min: 30 mg SC q24h (can consider 40 mg SC q24h if >100 kg and BMI >40).
[c]Contraindicated if weight <50 kg or CrCl <30. Use with caution if CrCl 30-50.

TABLE 18-6	VENOUS THROMBOEMBOLISM (VTE) TREATMENT OPTIONS
First-Line Therapy	**Alternative**
Enoxaparin: 1 mg/kg SC q12h. Adjust for extremes of weight and renal dysfunction. See text for prescribing details.	• IV UFH: see Table 18-2. • Enoxaparin: 1.5 mg/kg SC q24h (renally adjusted). • Rivaroxaban: 15 mg PO bid with food for 3 wk followed by 20 mg PO qday with food. Not recommended for CrCl <30 mL/min or on dialysis. • Apixaban: 10 mg PO bid for 7 d, and then 5 mg PO bid for 6 mo. Dosage adjustments in the presence of drug interactions and liver dysfunction. • Dabigatran: 150 mg PO bid. Not recommended for CrCl <30 mL/min.

For bridge therapy with enoxaparin/heparin administration ONLY: Initiate warfarin therapy together and continue enoxaparin/heparin for at least 5 d and until INR ≥2 for at least 24 h. Prolonged or lifelong therapy should be considered for all patients with unprovoked VTE (DVT and/or PE) and patients with recurrent DVT or PE.

UFH, unfractionated heparin; CrCl, creatinine clearance; INR, international normalized ratio; DVT, deep venous thrombosis; PE, pulmonary embolism.

Secondary Stroke Prevention
See Table 18-8 for secondary stroke prevention options.

TREATMENT OF HIGH INTERNATIONAL NORMALIZED RATIO

- **Treatment must be individualized!**
- There's sort of and then there's REALLY BLEEDING TO DEATH.
- Vitamin K can be given in equivalent dosages PO or IVPB. Subcutaneous administration is not recommended because of unpredictable response.
- Oral administration is preferred for minor bleeding. IV administration should be reserved for major bleeding.

TABLE 18-7	HEART VALVE REPLACEMENT TREATMENT OPTIONS	
Type	**First-Line Therapy**	**Alternative**
Bioprosthetic	• Mitral: warfarin, INR 2-3 for 3 mo, and then change to ASA 81 mg q24h.[a] • Aortic: ASA 81 mg PO q24h.[a] • Patient with a history of systemic embolism or known atrial thrombus: warfarin INR 2-3 for at least 3 mo or until clot resolution is documented.	Warfarin: INR 2-3 long-term with bioprosthetic valves and additional risk factors including atrial fibrillation, hypercoagulable state, or low ejection fraction.
	If there is a history of atherosclerotic vascular disease and no contraindications, add ASA 81 mg PO qday to warfarin.	
Mechanical	• Bileaflet or tilting disk in aortic position: warfarin INR 2-3. • All others or bileaflet or tilting disk in mitral position: warfarin INR 2.5-3.5.	Warfarin: INR 2.5-3.5 for any with risk factors for thromboembolism (atrial fibrillation, anterior apical STEMI, left atrial enlargement, hypercoagulable state, low ejection fraction).
	If no contraindications present, addition of ASA 81 mg PO qday if atrial fibrillation, hypercoagulable state, low ejection fraction, or a history of atherosclerotic vascular disease.	

INR, international normalized ratio; STEMI, ST-elevation myocardial infarction.
[a]ASA 75-100 mg has a similar efficacy yet lower bleeding risk than higher daily doses. In combination with clopidogrel, ASA <100 mg/d has been associated with lower bleeding risk.

TABLE 18-8	SECONDARY STROKE PREVENTION OPTIONS	
Stroke Type	First-Line Therapy	Alternative
Ischemic	Duration: lifelong (choose one): • ASA 81 mg PO qday[a] • Clopidogrel 75 mg PO qday • ASA 25-dipyrid-amole 200 mg PO bid	Cilostazol 100 mg PO bid
Cardioembolic stroke, mitral stenosis, or atrial fibrillation	Choose one: • Warfarin: INR 2-3 • Dabigatran: 150 mg PO bid, renally adjusted • Rivaroxaban: 20 mg PO qday, renally adjusted • Apixaban: 5 mg PO bid. Adjusted for kidney/hepatic function, body weight, age, and the presence of drug interactions • ASA 81 mg PO qday plus clopidogrel 75 mg qday if warfarin is avoided for reasons other than bleeding[a]	

[a]ASA 75-100 mg has a similar efficacy yet lower bleeding risk than higher daily doses. In combination with clopidogrel, ASA <100 mg/d has been associated with lower bleeding risk.

• If vitamin K is given IVPB, administer slowly to minimize risk of anaphylactoid reaction.
• The onset of action of oral vitamin K is 6 to 12 hours and 1 to 2 hours for IV. The peak effect is in 24 to 48 hours and 12 to 14 hours, respectively.
• Vitamin K is not recommended in the following circumstances:
    • INR <4.5 with no active bleeding, with and no surgery or procedure planned within 24 hours.
    • INR ≥4.5 and <9 with no risk factors for bleeding or falling, with and no surgery or procedure planned within 24 hours.

TABLE 18-9	WARFARIN REVERSAL: WITHOUT BLEEDING	
Situation	INR	Treatment
No planned surgical intervention within 24 h	<4.5	Lower or hold 1 dose of warfarin; monitor
	4.5-9 PLUS additional risk factors for bleeding	Hold warfarin + phytonadione 2.5 mg PO
	4.5-9 with NO additional bleeding risk factors	Hold 1-2 doses of warfarin; monitor
	>9	Hold warfarin + phytonadione 2.5 or 5 mg PO
Pending intervention within 24 h	<4.5	Hold warfarin + phytonadione 2.5 mg PO or IV May consider additional doses if INR remains elevated after 12 h
	≥4.5	Hold warfarin + phytonadione 5 mg PO or IV May consider additional doses if INR remains elevated after 12 h
Urgent or emergent surgery/ procedure	Any	See text, "Warfarin: Life-Threatening Bleeding or Need for Emergent Surgical Procedure"

Warfarin Reversal: Without Bleeding

Please see Table 18-9 for warfarin reversal without bleeding.

Warfarin Reversal: Minor Bleed

Please see Figure 18-1 for algorithm for warfarin reversal with minor bleeding.

Warfarin Reversal: Major, Non–Life-Threatening Bleeding

- Please see Figure 18-2 for algorithm for warfarin reversal with major, *non*–life-threatening bleeding.

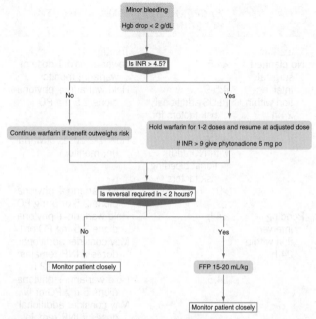

Figure 18-1. Warfarin reversal with minor bleeding. INR, international normalized ratio; FFP, fresh frozen plasma. (From Casabar E, Portell J, eds. *Barnes-Jewish Hospital Tool Book.* Department of Pharmacy, Barnes-Jewish Hospital, 2017, with permission.)

- Prothrombin complex concentrate (PCC) (Kcentra) includes 4 factors: II, VII, IX, and X; and proteins C and S.
- Uses of PCC (Kcentra) include the following:
  - Warfarin-associated life-threatening bleeding
  - Warfarin-associated major, <u>non</u>–life-threatening bleeding with INR >6
  - Warfarin-associated major bleeding with volume overload
  - Warfarin reversal for emergent surgical procedure
  - Can be considered for rivaroxaban- or apixaban-associated life-threatening bleeding
- Please see Table 18-10 for dosing of Kcentra.

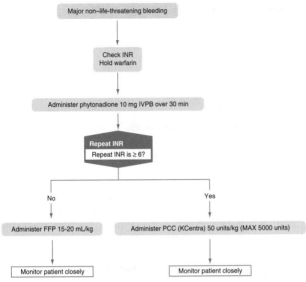

Figure 18-2. Warfarin reversal: major, *non*–life-threatening bleeding. INR, international normalized ratio; FFP, fresh frozen plasma; PCC, prothrombin complex concentrate. (From Casabar E, Portell J, eds. *Barnes-Jewish Hospital Tool Book.* Department of Pharmacy, Barnes-Jewish Hospital, 2017, with permission.)

TABLE 18-10	KCENTRA DOSING
INR	**Dose**
<2-3.9	25 units/kg (max 2500 units)
4-6	35 units/kg (max 3500 units)
>6	50 units/kg (max 5000 units)

INR, international normalized ratio.

Warfarin: Life-Threatening Bleeding or Need for Emergent Surgical Procedure

- Please see Figure 18-3 for algorithm for warfarin reversal with major, life-threatening bleeding.
- Life-threatening bleeding, any of the following:
  - Intracerebral bleeding
  - Uncontrolled gastrointestinal bleeding

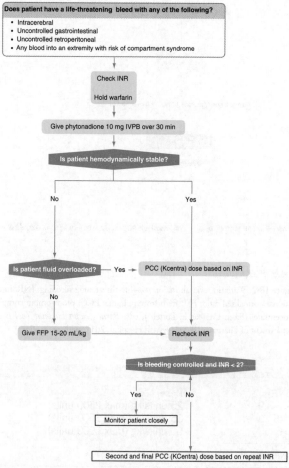

Figure 18-3. Warfarin reversal: major, life-threatening bleeding. INR, international normalized ratio; PCC, prothrombin complex concentrate; FFP, fresh frozen plasma. (From Casabar E, Portell J, eds. *Barnes-Jewish Hospital Tool Book.* Department of Pharmacy, Barnes-Jewish Hospital, 2017, with permission.)

- Uncontrolled retroperitoneal bleeding
- Any bleeding into an extremity with risk of compartment syndrome
- Or if emergent surgical intervention needed within 60 minutes
- Other recommendations
  - Identify the source and cause of bleed.
  - Evaluate aPTT, PT/INR, hemoglobin and hematocrit, platelets, electrolytes, ±fibrinogen.
  - Therapeutic ranges for monitoring warfarin (PT/INR), heparin (aPTT, anti-Xa), or LMWH (anti-Xa) must not be applied to the direct thrombin inhibitors or Factor Xa inhibitors.
  - Institute supportive strategies by means of discontinuation of anticoagulant, mechanical compression, administration of blood products, fluid resuscitation, and hemodynamic/respiratory support.
  - Maintain normal body temperature, blood pH, and electrolyte balance (e.g., Ca^{2+}) to facilitate coagulation.
  - If applicable, apply packing or dressing, and use local hemostatic measures or surgical intervention to control bleeding.
  - After major bleeding is controlled and the patient is stabilized, reassess the patient for risk of thromboembolism and initiate a short-acting agent if anticoagulation is required.

Heparin Reversal

Protamine 1 mg for each 100 units of heparin administered in the last 2 hours (maximum dose 50 mg).

Enoxaparin Reversal

Please see Figure 18-4 for enoxaparin reversal.

Direct Thrombin Inhibitor Reversal

Please see Figure 18-5 for direct thrombin inhibitor reversal algorithm.

Factor Xa Inhibitor Reversal

Please see Figure 18-6 for Factor Xa Inhibitor reversal algorithm.

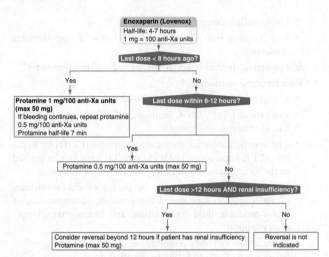

Figure 18-4. Enoxaparin reversal algorithm. (From Casabar E, Portell J, eds. *Barnes-Jewish Hospital Tool Book*. Department of Pharmacy, Barnes-Jewish Hospital, 2017, with permission.)

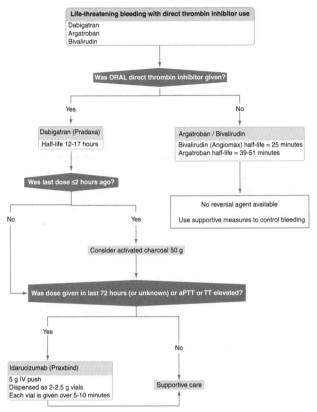

Figure 18-5. Direct thrombin inhibitor reversal algorithm. aPTT, activated partial thromboplastin time; TT, thrombin time. (From Casabar E, Portell J, eds. *Barnes-Jewish Hospital Tool Book*. Department of Pharmacy, Barnes-Jewish Hospital, 2017, with permission.)

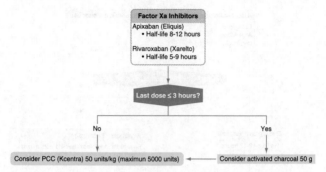

Figure 18-6. Factor Xa inhibitor reversal algorithm. PCC, prothrombin complex concentrate. (From Casabar E, Portell J, eds. *Barnes-Jewish Hospital Tool Book*. Department of Pharmacy, Barnes-Jewish Hospital, 2017, with permission.)

19

Approach to Consultation

Kirsten Dunn, Thomas M. Ciesielski, and
Thomas M. De Fer

TIPS FOR CALLING A CONSULT

Calling for a consultation from another service is a skill that needs to be developed, and calling with incomplete information may lead to significant frustration for the primary service and the consulting service. The house staff safety and quality council at Barnes-Jewish Hospital and Washington University developed a mnemonic for appropriately calling a consult, from a framework developed in emergency medicine.[1]

A. Approach

Preparation: See and examine the patient and review pertinent clinical information.

Contact: Introduce yourself and your service.

Information: Provide basic patient information including name, date of birth, location, and attending requesting consultation.

B. Background and basic question

Background: **Brief** one-liner about the patient, including age, gender, relevant medical history.

Basic question/concern: "We are consulting you for _____." My attending told me to call you is not an appropriate consultation question!

C. Communicate

Agree upon urgency. The service being consulted may be more experienced in the issue but has a disadvantage in having not yet seen this particular patient.

Any immediate recommendations? Like preliminary diagnostic tests.

Call back information with name(s), number(s), and expected timeframe.

10 COMMANDMENTS OF CONSULTATION

Guiding principles for providing effective medicine consultations were first suggested by Goldman and colleagues in 1983.[2]

The commandments of consultation remain relevant today, although they were updated and slightly modified in 2006.[3] A meshing of the two lists and are presented:

1. **Determine the question being asked and who the customer is.** As a guiding principle, and when taking the initial phone call from the requesting service, always determine the specific question he/she wants to be answered—if the question is not entirely clear they may be asking for co-management (particularly on surgical services). Clarifying the question and expectations will be helpful, especially in situations in which the patient has an extensive and complicated medical history. Thus, a typical consultation note should begin by stating a specific problem, such as "Called to see this 78-year-old woman with type 2 diabetes and hypertension for perioperative glucose control …."

2. **Establish urgency.** Always determine if the consult is emergent, urgent, or elective, and let the primary service know when they can expect your recommendations on the basis of this assessment or urgency.

3. **Look for yourself.** Seldom do the answers to the consultation question lie in the chart; more often than not, independent data gathering is required, including reviewing prior admissions or getting further testing. In many cases, the data review combined with a complete history and physical exam from an internal medicine perspective will establish the diagnosis and guide a treatment plan.

4. **Be as brief as appropriate.** It is not necessary to repeat the details and data already in the primary team's note; obviously, as much new data independently gathered should be recorded.

5. **Be specific, thorough, and assist when requested.** Try to be goal-oriented and keep the discussion and differential diagnosis concise. When recommending drugs, always include dose, frequency, and route. It is appropriate to ask if the requesting provider would like orders put in on their patient.

6. **Provide contingency plans, and how to execute those plans.** Try to anticipate potential problems (e.g., if using escalating doses of a β-blocker for rapid atrial fibrillation, make sure that regular BP checks are instituted). Staff (nursing/ancillary) on other floors may not be used to treating patients with problems outside of the floor's specialty. Clarify who can be contacted after-hours for additional help.

7. **Discuss "turf" with the requesting provider.** Discuss with the requesting physician if the expectation is co-management of the patient or answering one specific question.

8. **Pragmatically teach with tact.** Share your insights and expertise without condescension, but make it appropriate to others' level of training, specialty, and the clinical situation.

9. **Talk is cheap, and effective, and essential.** Communicate your recommendations directly to the requesting physician. There is no substitute for direct personal contact.

10. **Appropriately follow up, usually daily.** Suggestions are more likely to be translated into orders when the consultant continues to follow up. If the problem is no longer active, the consultant may sign off, although this should be discussed with the requesting physician in advance.

References

1. Kessler CS, Tadisina KK, Saks M. The 5Cs of consultation: training medical students to communicate effectively in the emergency department. *J Emerg Med* 2015;9:713-21.

2. Goldman L, Lee T, Rudd P. Ten commandments for effective consultations. *Arch Intern Med* 1983;143:1753-55.

3. Salerno SM, Hurst FP, Halvorson S, Mercado DL. Principles of effective consultation: an update for the 21st-century consultant. *Arch Intern Med* 2007;167:271-75.

Preoperative Cardiovascular Risk Assessment

20

Thomas M. De Fer

- Preoperative cardiovascular evaluation is aimed at eliminating or treating risk factors to reduce the risk of significant adverse cardiac events (e.g., myocardial infarction [MI], unstable angina, heart failure [HF], arrhythmia, and death). No patient is ever "cleared" for surgery. We can really only estimate risk and this is often annoying to our surgical colleagues.

- Some procedures are known to be associated with inherently low risk (<1%) for major adverse cardiac events (MI or death).[1] **Low-risk procedures** include endoscopy, cataract/glaucoma surgery, plastic/dermatologic and other superficial procedures, and breast surgery. In this circumstance, preprocedure evaluation (including ECG and so-called routine labs) is of very limited value in asymptomatic patients.

- Risk assessment guidelines have been published by the American College of Cardiology/American Heart Association (ACC/AHA) Task Force.[1] History, physical examination, and ECG are important components of a thorough clinical assessment and help determine the extent of diagnostic testing required.

- Many common arrhythmias are not a clear contraindication to surgery. Well, OK, sustained V-tach and complete heart block are. Call for help! Atrial fibrillation is generally not a contraindication, although the matter of anticoagulation must be considered carefully. The patient's cardiologist should be consulted regarding pacemakers and defibrillators.

- Patients who meet current clinical practice guidelines for intervention for moderate to severe valvular stenosis/regurgitation should have this addressed prior to elective surgery.

- The **ACC/AHA algorithm for preoperative cardiac risk assessment** is detailed in Figure 20-1.[1]

- An **emergency procedure** is defined as one where a life or limb is threatened if it does not occur within <6 hours.[1] It is not unusual for the term "emergency" to be used very imprecisely, so be mindful of this. In very few circumstances is a hip fracture repair an actual emergency.

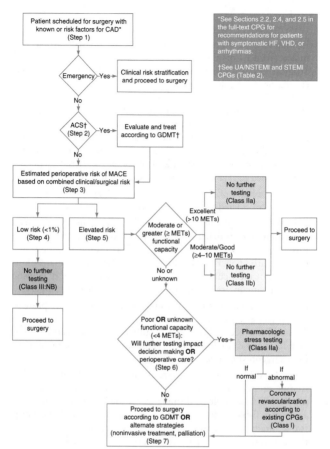

Figure 20-1. 2014 ACC/AHA algorithm for perioperative cardiac assessment. Table 2 refers to Table 2 in the published reference. Class I, strong recommendation regarding benefit; Class IIa, intermediate strength recommendation regarding benefit; Class IIb, weak recommendation, marginal benefit-risk ratio; Class III:NB, strong recommendation against, no benefit. CAD, coronary artery disease; CPG, clinical practice guideline; HF, heart failure; VHD, valvular heart disease; UA, unstable angina; NSTEMI, non-ST-elevation myocardial infarction; STEMI, ST-elevation myocardial infarction; ACS, acute coronary syndrome; GDMT, guideline-directed medical therapy; MACE, major adverse cardiac event; METS, metabolic equivalents. (From Fleisher LA, Fleischmann KE, Auerbach AD, et al. 2014 ACC/AHA guideline on perioperative cardiovascular evaluation and management of patients undergoing noncardiac surgery: a report of the American College of Cardiology/American Heart Association Task Force on Practice Guidelines. *Circulation* 2014;130:e278-333, with permission.)

- Perioperative risk may be assessed with the **revised cardiac risk index (RCRI)** or the American College of Surgery **National Surgical Quality Improvement Program (NSQIP) universal risk calculator.**[2,3] The RCRI risk factors are coronary artery disease (CAD), HF, cerebrovascular disease, diabetes requiring insulin, chronic kidney disease (creatinine [Cr] >2.0 mg/dL), and high-risk surgery (e.g., open intraperitoneal or intrathoracic and vascular procedures). The presence of more than one risk factor conveys a risk of major cardiac complications of >1%. The NSQIP calculator is available online at https://riskcalculator.facs.org/RiskCalculator/ (last accessed 2/5/18). Honestly, it's really neat, you should try it.

- Climbing a flight of stairs or walking up a hill at a normal pace are generally considered to be about 4 METS (metabolic equivalents).

- Do not perform preoperative noninvasive testing until you've very, very carefully considered what you will do if it happens to be positive. If the answer is nothing, well… This DOES include stable patients with known CAD (with or without prior revascularization) who do not meet current clinical practice guidelines for diagnostic or therapeutic interventions, irrespective of the planned surgery.

- Performing a **percutaneous coronary intervention** (PCI) prior to noncardiac elective surgery is a complex and controversial issue. This will not occur (better not occur!) without the learned input of at least one cardiologist. PCI is absolutely not a cure for all your (or a surgeon's) preoperative anxieties.

- **β-Blockers:** Oh how things have changed. Multiple prior smaller studies supported the use of perioperative β-blockade; however, the POISE trial, while confirming a decrease in cardiac events with aggressive β-blockade, showed an increase in overall mortality, stroke, bradycardia, and hypotension.[4] Systematic reviews support this conclusion.[5] If the patient has been on a β-blocker as a part of his/her routine medication regimen, it should simply be continued. β-Blocker therapy may be appropriate for those patients with intermediate- to high-risk ischemia on preoperative stress testing, but the risk of stroke and other contraindications should be carefully considered. β-Blockers may also be reasonable for patients with ≥3 RCRI risk factors.[1,2] If β-blocker therapy is opted for, it should be started at least more than one day in advance to assess tolerability and safety. β-Blockade should NOT be started on the day of surgery.[1]

- **Antiplatelet therapy:** The POISE-2 trial results do not support the routine perioperative initiation of aspirin in patients at risk for CAD.[6] The risk-to-benefit ratio of discontinuing aspirin and/or P2Y$_{12}$ receptor blocker (e.g., clopidogrel, prasugrel, ticagrelor) in patients who have had stenting is a far more complicated matter, particularly in those who have not completed the minimum duration of dual antiplatelet therapy (30 d for a bare metal stent and 6 mo for a drug-eluting stent). In such cases, a cardiology consultation should be obtained. No one reading this book should make that decision on their own!

- Patients on long-term statin, angiotensin converting enzyme inhibitor, and/or calcium channel blocker therapy should continue these medications during the perioperative period. Statins may be initiated perioperatively in those for whom it is indicated.

- Continuation of preoperative antihypertensive treatment throughout the perioperative period is critical, particularly if the patient is on clonidine (risk of rebound hypertension). Consider switching the patient to IV or transdermal formulations of medications if the patient will be NPO for an extended period.

References

1. Fleisher LA, Fleischmann KE, Auerbach AD, et al. 2014 ACC/AHA guideline on perioperative cardiovascular evaluation and management of patients undergoing noncardiac surgery: a report of the American College of Cardiology/ American Heart Association Task Force on Practice Guidelines. *Circulation* 2014;130:e278-333.
2. Lee TH, Marcantonio ER, Mangione CM, et al. Derivation and prospective validation of a simple index for prediction of cardiac risk of major noncardiac surgery. *Circulation* 1999;100:1043-9.
3. Cohen ME, Ko CY, Bilimoria KY, et al. Development and validation of a risk calculator for prediction of cardiac risk after surgery. *Circulation* 2011;124:381-7.
4. POISE Study Group. Effects of extended-release metoprolol succinate in patients undergoing non-cardiac surgery (POISE trial): a randomised controlled trial. *Lancet* 2008;371:1839-47.
5. Wijeysundera DD, Nkonde-Price C, et al. Perioperative beta blockade in noncardiac surgery: a systematic review for the 2014 ACC/AHA guideline on perioperative cardiovascular evaluation and management of patients undergoing noncardiac surgery: a report of the American College of Cardiology/ American Heart Association Task Force on Practice Guidelines. *Circulation* 2014;130:2246-64.
6. Devereaux PJ, Mrkobrada M, Sessler DI, et al. Aspirin in patients undergoing noncardiac surgery. *N Engl J Med* 2014;370:1494-503.

Dermatology

21

Caroline Morris and Kara Sternhell-Blackwell

The intern's guide to dermatology consults because not every rash is "maculopapular." Except when it is. And even then, the dermatologists will admonish you for saying so. That's just the rule.

TOXIC EPIDERMAL NECROLYSIS

- **Toxic epidermal necrolysis (TEN) is a true dermatology emergency** (contrary to popular belief—this is not always an oxymoron)! **Consult dermatology immediately.** Yes, even if it is 3:00 a.m. Seriously!
- **Think about TEN if you see blisters/erosions, skin pain, and mucosal involvement.**
- TEN and Stevens-Johnson syndrome (SJS) are two rare and potentially fatal mucocutaneous adverse drug reactions characterized by extensive erythema, necrosis, and exfoliation.
- **History**
  - Drug history: **Drugs are almost always the inciting cause.** TEN typically occurs within the first 8 weeks of therapy. The most common offenders include sulfonamides, anticonvulsants, antibiotics, NSAIDs, antiretrovirals, and allopurinol. Less than 5% of patients report no history of medication use.
  - Typical symptoms consist of a prodrome of upper respiratory tract symptoms, fever, and painful skin.
- **Physical examination**: fever, painful erythema of skin, blisters and/or erosions, mucosal erosions, and conjunctival erythema. Diagnosis requires involvement of two or more mucosal surfaces. The skin eruption is usually painful, a useful key in making the diagnosis. Degree of skin involvement: 10% = SJS, 10% to 30% = SJS-TEN overlap, >30% = TEN.
- **Evaluation**: complete blood count (CBC), complete metabolic panel (CMP), if there is respiratory distress a chest radiograph (CXR), and skin biopsy
- **Treatment**
  - **Stop suspect drug(s) and all other nonessential medications!**
  - Admit to an ICU.

- IV fluids, nasogastric tube
- Sterile protocol, antiseptic solution, non-adherent dressings. Dermatology should provide wound care instruction guides.
- Pain control
- Antibiotics if high suspicion for sepsis
- **Systemic steroids and/or intravenous immunoglobulins (IVIG) 1 g/kg × 3 or 4 days** (decided on a case-by-case basis)
- Ophthalmology consultation for all TEN patients
- Gynecology consultation for vaginal involvement; urology consultation for urethral involvement

- **Clinical pearls:** Hepatitis occurs in 10% of patients. Most patients have anemia and lymphopenia. Neutropenia is associated with poor prognosis. Hypothermia is more indicative of sepsis than fever. Patients with HIV, systemic lupus, or a bone marrow transplant are at higher risk of developing TEN.
- **Prognosis:** TEN has a frightfully high mortality rate of 30% to 40%, which is most often secondary to sepsis, renal failure due to hypovolemic shock, or acute respiratory distress syndrome.

TOXIC SHOCK SYNDROME

- **Toxic shock syndrome (TSS) is an emergency. Consult infectious diseases immediately!**
- **Think about TSS if you see: sick patient, diffuse rash, recent surgery, or menses.**
- TSS is caused by toxic shock syndrome toxin-1 (TSST-1) and other enterotoxins released by *Staphylococcus aureus* and *Streptococcus pyogenes.* These toxins cause overstimulation of many immune processes leading to serious illness.
- **History:** Age, immunocompromised status, menstrual history, recent surgeries, diabetes, chronic cardiac or pulmonary disease. Typically, the patient has a painful erythematous skin eruption, sudden onset high fever, nausea/vomiting, diarrhea, sore throat, confusion, headache, myalgias, and hypotension.
- **Physical examination:** High fever, erythematous rash initially appearing on trunk and then spreading to arms and legs with involvement of the palms and soles, ultimately progressing to diffuse erythema and edema. Typically involves the oral mucosa. In 10 to 12 days, there is desquamation of the top layer of the epidermis (as opposed to full thickness seen in TEN).

- **Evaluation**: Blood cultures, CBC (leukocytosis), CMP (hyponatremia, hypokalemia, hypocalcemia, elevated LFTs [liver function tests]), ECG (arrhythmias), CXR. Consider: serologic testing for Rocky Mountain spotted fever, leptospirosis, measles, hepatitis B surface antigen, antinuclear antibody (ANA), venereal disease research laboratory test, monospot antibody, rapid strep test, lumbar puncture (should be normal).

- **Diagnosis**: usually clinical with the constellation of symptoms including fever, typical rash, hypotension, multiorgan involvement

- **Treatment**
  - **Remove any infected foreign bodies!**
  - Empiric IV antibiotics against *Streptococcus* and *Staphylococcus*, IV clindamycin + IV vancomycin; tailor therapy to culture results.
  - Aggressive IV fluid repletion
  - Consider IVIG.
  - Monitor carefully for hypotension/shock.

- **Clinical pearls**: Staphylococcal scalded skin syndrome has a similar clinical picture; however, it generally occurs in immunocompromised adults. *S. aureus* is the most common cause of TSS; however, exotoxin-producing streptococci can result in a similar clinical picture with higher mortality. Clindamycin suppresses synthesis of TSST-1, while β-lactamase-resistant antibiotics may increase its synthesis and, therefore, clindamycin should be included in the antibiotic regimen.

NECROTIZING FASCIITIS

- **This is an emergency! Consult surgery immediately.** Also refer to the "Necrotizing Soft Tissues Infections" section in Chapter 28, General Surgery.

- Think about necrotizing fasciitis if you see rapidly progressive red, purple or dusky and foul-smelling skin wound, sometimes with "dishwasher gray" drainage, and severe pain.

- Necrotizing soft tissue infections can be divided into two distinct bacteriologic categories: type I (polymicrobial) and type II (group A streptococcal).

- **History**: Recent surgical or traumatic wound with rapid progression. Typically the involved area becomes erythematous, indurated, and severely painful. Pain out of proportion to physical exam findings is often a clue.

- **Physical examination**: Within hours the involved area can become dusky blue to black, indicating necrosis. Crepitus may be present because of formation of subcutaneous gas. Altered mental status may occur.
- **Evaluation**: Blood cultures, creatine kinase (CK), plain films for soft tissue gas, non-contrast CT. Hyponatremia, neutrophilia, or leukopenia may be seen.
- **Treatment**
  - Wide surgical debridement and tissue culture. All necrosis must go!
  - Empiric IV antibiotics effective against streptococci, anaerobes, methicillin-resistant *Staphylococcus aureus* (MRSA), and gram-negative bacilli. Include clindamycin for antitoxin effect.
- **Clinical pearls**: Time is essential, call for surgical help immediately! Mortality rate is as high as 25%.

PEMPHIGUS VULGARIS AND BULLOUS PEMPHIGOID

- Pemphigus vulgaris (PV) and bullous pemphigoid (BP) require urgent dermatology consults.
- Pemphigus and pemphigoid are a group of rare, potentially fatal, autoimmune blistering diseases caused by autoantibodies directed against structural proteins of the skin, resulting in mucosal and cutaneous intraepithelial blisters. Almost all patients with PV have mucosal involvement. BP tends to affect elderly patients more often and may be preceded by weeks to months of a prodromal phase.
- **History**: flaccid bullae and erosions with mucosal involvement (PV) and pruritus with tense bullae in an elderly person (BP)
- **Physical examination**: flaccid or tense bullae, percentage of body surface area (BSA) involved, mucosal involvement
- **Evaluation**: Skin biopsy with direct immunofluorescence. Enzyme-linked immunosorbent assay for desmoglein 1,3 and/or bullous pemphigoid antigen 1 (BPАg1, a.k.a., BP230), and bullous pemphigoid antigen 2 (BPАg2, a.k.a., BP180). Well doesn't that sound fancy!
- **Treatment**
  - PV: steroids, rituximab, mycophenolate mofetil, azathioprine
  - BP: steroids (topical or systemic), tetracycline, azathioprine, dapsone, mycophenolate mofetil, rituximab
  - Of course, all of that is above any intern's pay grade.

- **Clinical pearls**: PV is associated with a higher mortality than BP; thus, PV requires more aggressive treatment. Early, aggressive treatment is associated with better outcomes. Most patients do not require hospitalization unless infected, high BSA affected, or having difficulty in maintaining fluid balance. Other etiologies of blistering diseases include infectious, autoimmune, allergic hypersensitivity, metabolic, paraneoplastic, and genetic.

VASCULITIS

- Another perfectly good reason to consult dermatology.
- Vasculitis is due to inflammatory leukocytes within the vessel wall leading to reactive damage of the mural structures causing loss of vessel integrity and may result in downstream ischemia and necrosis.
- **History**: Drug history, history of connective tissue disease, malignancy, or infection. Skin findings may be itchy, painful, or asymptomatic.
- **Physical examination**: **palpable purpura** (raised, nonblanchable lesions that may blister or ulcerate) on the lower extremities or dependent areas
- **Evaluation**: CBC, CMP, urinalysis (UA), skin biopsy; if concerned for systemic disease, then consider: CXR, throat culture for strep, erythrocyte sedimentation rate, hepatitis panel, cryoglobulins, ANA, rheumatoid factor, antiphospholipid antibody, antineutrophil cytoplasmic antibodies, serum protein electrophoresis (SPEP).
- **Diagnosis**: Skin biopsy; concern for systemic involvement if fever, arthralgias, abdominal pain, pulmonary symptoms, hematuria, or proteinuria
- **Treatment**
  - Discontinue potential causative drug(s). Most common culprits include aspirin, sulfonamides, penicillin, barbiturates, amphetamines, and propylthiouracil.
  - Treat underlying disorder(s) (i.e., infection, malignancy, or connective tissue disease).
  - Antihistamines, NSAIDs, colchicine, dapsone, antimalarials. Yes, some of that sounds like mumbo jumbo.
  - If systemic involvement, prednisone, azathioprine, cyclophosphamide, IVIG, plasmapheresis can be used.
- **Clinical pearls**: Up to 50% of cases are idiopathic. Common causes of vasculitis include drugs, infection, connective tissue disease, and malignancy. Thrombocytopenia is associated with

nonpalpable purpura. Disseminated intravascular coagulation and warfarin necrosis cause extensive purpura. *Neisseria* sepsis and Rocky Mountain spotted fever also cause petechiae and purpura. Acral hemorrhagic papules, pustules, or vesicles may result from thrombi or septic emboli.

DRUG HYPERSENSITIVITY SYNDROME (SEVERE DRUG REACTION)

- This is grounds for an urgent dermatology consult.
- Drug-induced hypersensitivity syndrome (DHS) or drug reaction with eosinophilia and systemic symptoms (DRESS) is a rare but potentially fatal drug-induced hypersensitivity reaction that involves maculopapular (yep, this one has it!) skin eruption, hematologic abnormalities (eosinophilia, atypical lymphocytes), lymphadenopathy, and multiorgan manifestations (liver, renal, and lung most commonly).
- **History:** Drug history (sulfonamides, anticonvulsants, allopurinol, vancomycin, minocycline, dapsone). The history includes fever, rash, swelling, and lymphadenopathy.
- **Physical examination**
  - The rash is blanchable erythematous macules or exfoliative dermatitis.
  - Edema of the face, hands, and feet is seen.
  - Fever
  - Lymphadenopathy and hepatosplenomegaly may be present.
- **Evaluation:** CBC with differential (eosinophil count), CMP, UA, CXR
- **Treatment**
  - **Stop offending drug!**
  - Systemic steroids (often requires long duration taper), symptomatic management with topical steroids and antihistamines.
  - Order CBC with diff and CMP every day the patient is in-house.
- **Clinical pearls:** DRESS typically develops within 8 weeks of starting the causative drug. Up to 50% will develop fulminant hepatic necrosis if the drug is not stopped early in the course. Some anticonvulsants cross-react in 70% to 80% of patients (i.e., phenytoin, carbamazepine, and phenobarbital; valproic acid does not cross-react). There is a hereditary component and so patients should warn first-degree relatives that they may also be at high risk for a reaction. Recent viral infection may be a risk factor for worse disease course. Check thyroid-stimulating hormone 12 weeks after diagnosis as hypothyroidism can result from DHS.

ERYTHRODERMA (GENERALIZED EXFOLIATIVE DERMATITIS)

- Urgent dermatology consultation.
- Erythroderma, also known as exfoliative dermatitis, is a severe and potentially fatal condition that presents with diffuse erythema and scaling involving majority of the skin surface area. It is a clinical presentation of a broad spectrum of cutaneous and systemic diseases, drug hypersensitivity reactions, and more rarely Sézary syndrome.
- Most common causes: idiopathic, drug reaction, lymphoma and leukemia (including cutaneous T-cell lymphoma), atopic dermatitis (eczema), psoriasis, contact dermatitis
- **History:** prior skin disorder, drug history, duration of symptoms
- **Physical examination:** diffuse erythema of skin leading to exfoliative dermatitis, pruritus, keratoderma (thickening of the palms and soles), shivering/chills, alopecia
- **Evaluation:** CBC, CMP, SPEP, peripheral blood smear for Sézary cells, flow cytometry. Skin biopsy often demonstrates nonspecific findings.
- **Treatment**
  - Treat underlying skin condition, if known (i.e., psoriasis, eczema).
  - Discontinue any suspect drugs.
  - Search for and treat underlying malignancy.
  - Topical steroid ointment "soak and smear" (soaking the affected body part or whole body by bathing in plain water for 20 min, immediately [without drying the skin] followed by smearing the ointment over the affected area), emollients, and systemic antihistamines.
  - Monitor closely for electrolyte and fluid imbalances, high-output cardiac failure, renal failure, sepsis, and hypothermia.
- **Clinical pearls:** 25% to 30% of cases are idiopathic. The course and prognosis depend on the underlying etiology. A diligent search for the underlying cause is often required. Most patients do not require hospitalization unless infected.

Neurology

Asher Albertson and Renee van Stavern

STROKE

- Strokes frequently occur on the inpatient service. Your patients have atrial fibrillation, endocarditis, hypertension, and vascular disease, all of which are ingredients for an anxiety-inducing late-night page about an acute change in the neurologic exam. Your response in the first few moments is critical. Time is brain!

- Stroke is divided into two broad categories: **ischemic** (usually involving decreased blood flow to a distinct cerebral vascular territory) and **hemorrhagic** (involving bleeding into the brain). Management of course is vastly different but no less emergent in either case. It is important to remember that time is brain. Studies have shown repeatedly that delaying potential treatment even a few minutes may have a tremendous impact on functional recovery. So no pressure...

When Called for an Acute Neurologic Change Concerning for Stroke

- Immediately drop everything (that urgent order for a bowel regimen can wait) and see the patient. **Stroke is a neurologic emergency!**
- Obtain the vital signs and a finger stick glucose.
- Obtain a pertinent history.
  - What is the time course? Treatment decisions (tissue plasminogen activator [TPA] and thrombectomy) are based on the time last known or seen normal, not the time the patient was found by the nurse.
  - Is the patient on anticoagulation? Has he/she had recent major surgery?
  - Are there lab abnormalities or medications that could alter the neurologic exam or be a contraindication to treatment?
  - Were there signs or symptoms of a stroke mimic such as a seizure (although seizure sometimes occurs with stroke onset)?
  - Were there other associated signs and symptoms (thunderclap headache, nausea, or vomiting)?

- Perform a focused neurologic exam. The best thing to do is calculate the National Institutes of Health (NIH) stroke scale—this makes your life easy because it is a very focused neurologic exam and will be vital for treatment decisions. There are multiple apps as well as easy to print forms on the Web. The broad components are as follows:

  - Level of consciousness: Alert? Able to follow commands? Answer questions?
  - Gaze: Do they have gaze deviation or difficulty looking one direction?
  - Visual fields: Can they count fingers in all quadrants?
  - Facial palsy: Is there a facial droop?
  - Motor: Is there weakness in the arms or legs?
  - Ataxia: Is there difficulty with finger to nose testing?
  - Sensation: Can they feel equally on both sides?
  - Language: Can they name simple objects?
  - Dysarthria: Are they slurred?
  - Neglect: Can they recognize both sides equally?

- **Order a "critical-life threatening" head CT.** Do not wait for transport. Do not pass go. You may need to wheel the patient to radiology yourself (with help). If your index of suspicion is high enough based on the phone call, the CT can be ordered while speed walking to the patient's room. The exam/NIH stroke scale can be completed en route to the scanner.

- **If you suspect a stroke, activate the TPA pager.** The sooner the neurology service is involved in emergent stroke care, the better.

- Patients with a last known well within 4.5 hours may be eligible for thrombolytic therapy with TPA. While protocols differ by institution, absolute contraindications include blood on head CT, serious head trauma in the last 3 months, platelet count of <100,000/μL of blood, or therapeutic anticoagulation. Blood pressure >185/110 mm Hg must be corrected gently and blood glucose levels <50 or >400 mg/dL must also be corrected.

- There are multiple other relative contraindications, and the risks of these decisions must be taken in the context of a potential benefit to the patient. These include major surgery in the last 2 weeks, a history of intracranial hemorrhage, metastasis to the brain, seizure at onset, arterial puncture to a noncompressible site, large unsecured aneurysms, arteriovenous malformations, and recent gastrointestinal or genitourinary hemorrhage. These are best discussed in collaboration with the stroke team.

- This step may vary among institutions, so check your local protocol. After obtaining a head CT, patients with an NIH stroke scale of 6 or greater should receive a CT angiogram. This is to check for thrombi in the initial segment of the middle cerebral artery, the basilar artery, or the carotid artery. **Patients with one of these "large vessel occlusions" and a last known well within 7.3 hours are eligible for thrombectomy** (sometimes longer for basilar thrombosis). Clearly, this is not a decision anyone will let you make on your own. Thank goodness.
- **The possibility of thrombectomy should not deter the administration of TPA.**
- After receiving TPA or thrombectomy, patients should (ideally) be monitored in a specialized stroke unit or neurologic ICU and you should work with the stroke neurology team to facilitate transfer.
- Patients frequently present with so-called stroke mimics. These may include metabolic abnormalities such as hypoglycemia, hemiplegic migraine, or complex seizure. It is important to remember that migraine, metabolic abnormalities, and seizure can all occur coincidentally with a stroke and not to let these diminish your sense of urgency.
- While evaluating the patient (as if you didn't have enough on your plate), be sure to assess the patient's ability to protect their airway. All the TPA in the world won't help someone oxygenate.
- **If the patient's head CT shows intraparenchymal hemorrhage, please** do not **administer TPA.** Measure the size of the bleed and look for signs or swelling (loss of gray-white differentiation, sulcal effacement, or mid-line shift). The neurology service should be rapidly involved, and if the bleed is large, is associated with significant edema, or is in the posterior fossa, the neurosurgical service may need to be involved. The majority of these patients require rapid transfer to neurologic intensive care units. Meanwhile, check a coagulation panel and rapidly reverse any coagulopathy. Prothrombin complex concentrate is the fastest, most effective way to reverse patients with an elevated international normalized ratio (also the most expensive). Blood pressure should be controlled to a MAP goal of <110 mm Hg with IV labetalol if pulse rate >60, and IV hydralazine if it is not.
- After the initial acute ischemic stroke evaluation, make sure that these patients are receiving frequent neuro checks (at least q4h if on the floor). Any change in neurologic status should be followed by a stat head CT looking for hemorrhagic transformation. For the first 24 to 42 hours, stroke patients' blood pressure can be allowed to run higher. While protocols differ, if the patient did not receive TPA, treat for blood pressure >220/110 mm Hg. Patients who receive TPA need much tighter control for the first 24 hours (treat if >180/105 mm Hg).

- The next step is an evaluation of their risk factors for stroke.
  - Order an A1c and lipid panel, and start a high-intensity statin (atorvastatin or rosuvastatin) at the highest tolerated dose.
  - Order a carotid Doppler ultrasound or CT angiogram of the neck, unless the stroke is in the brainstem or cerebellum.
  - All patients with ischemic stroke should be started on an antiplatelet agent within 48 hours of arrival (typically aspirin).
  - Start anticoagulation in patients with atrial fibrillation/flutter at discharge and discontinue aspirin unless the patient has a cardiac indication for antiplatelet therapy plus anticoagulation.
  - Consider a Holter monitor or 30-day continuous loop recorder if no other obvious stroke etiology is discovered.

SEIZURE

- Seizures are frequently encountered on both inpatient and outpatient services. Remember that like late-night hospital cafeteria food, seizures come in many distressing shapes and sizes. While many seizures are generalized motor events, others are focal events and may vary widely in their level of cognitive involvement. Additionally, nonconvulsive or subclinical seizures occur relatively frequently, especially in critically ill patients.
- Seizures on the inpatient service occur for a variety of reasons. Patients with preexisting seizure disorders who miss medications (don't be careless with the med rec!) or develop an infection (lowers the seizure threshold) commonly present with breakthrough seizures. Toxic or metabolic abnormalities (e.g., alcohol, cocaine, amphetamines, hyper- or hypoglycemia, hyponatremia) are also common causes. Other important causes include vascular events (e.g., ischemic stroke, subarachnoid hemorrhage, intraparenchymal hemorrhage), new structural lesions (e.g., tumor, metastasis), or infections (e.g., meningitis, encephalitis).
- Any seizure lasting longer than 5 minutes or >1 seizure without a return to baseline is considered status epilepticus.

When Evaluating a Patient Who (May Have) Experienced a Single Seizure

- Make sure the patient has returned to their neurologic baseline.
- If this is their first seizure, order a head CT if not already done. You don't want to be that person who discharged someone with a new intracerebral mass.

- What were the features of the event: Were the eyes deviated? Was there symmetric jerking or arrhythmic, thrashing movements? How is the patient immediately after the event (awake, weak on one side, etc.)?

- Are there any obvious toxic or metabolic causes (e.g., illness, missed or added medications, recently stopped drinking)?

- Review all the patient's laboratory values looking for any abnormalities.

- Perform a thorough general and neurologic examination. Look for bruising or signs or trauma, especially on the sides of the tongue or cheeks. Check for any localizing or focal features in the cranial nerves and extremities.

- All patients with unprovoked first-time seizures need a brain MRI (ideally with fine sections through the temporal lobes). This will help assess for underlying structural causes such as a meningioma, cortical malformation, or tumor. Order a routine EEG, and consult a neurologist (either in the inpatient or outpatient setting, depending on the urgency).

- The majority of patients with unprovoked seizures who lack a clear underlying structural abnormality will not have a second seizure and do not warrant long-term antiepileptic drug therapy.

When Confronted with an Actively Seizing Patient

- First and foremost, don't panic! However, **status epilepticus is a neurologic emergency!**

- Make sure the airway is secure and the patient is hemodynamically stable. Do **NOT** insert objects into the patient's mouth (like your fingers). If safe, elevate the bedrails and roll the patient on his/her side. Administer facemask or nasal cannula oxygen if needed.

- Rapidly review the patient's laboratory values. If there have been no recent labs, order a STAT finger stick glucose, full chemistry panel, complete blood count, and toxicology screen.

- **Administer IV benzodiazepine**, lorazepam in 2 mg increments to a maximum dose of 0.1 mg/kg. Rectal diazepam (0.5 mg/kg with a max of 20 mg) or intramuscular midazolam (0.2 mg/kg) can be substituted if IV access is unavailable. Individual doses should be repeated until seizure activity abates. Stick with one drug. Never mix, never worry.

- If there is any chance the seizure is due to a metabolic cause or alcohol withdrawal, administer IV thiamine 100 mg followed by 50 mL of IV Dextrose 50%.

- **IV benzodiazepine therapy must be followed by administration of an IV antiepileptic.** Most guidelines recommend IV fosphenytoin at a dose of 15 mg/kg infused at a rate of 150 mg per hour. Alternative IV agents include valproic acid, levetiracetam, or lacosamide.
- If the patient continues to seize, then intubate, start an infusion of a midazolam or propofol titrated to seizure abatement, and transfer to an ICU with involvement of the neurology service and probable EEG monitoring.
- Order an urgent head CT when stable if a clear underlying cause is not immediately identified.
- Monitor the patient closely to assure a return to neurologic baseline. If they do not return to baseline, an EEG should be obtained to assess for nonconvulsive seizures. Remember that in the same way that a single ECG does not rule out atrial fibrillation, a 15-minute EEG does not rule out intermittent nonconvulsive seizures.
- All patients with prolonged seizures should have a creatinine kinase drawn to assess for rhabdomyolysis.

CENTRAL NERVOUS SYSTEM INFECTIONS

- Infections of the brain and spinal cord may involve the ventricles, the meninges, the parenchyma, or all of these.
- Bacterial meningitis typically presents as a rapidly progressive decline in mental status with multiple signs of acute infection.
- Viral meningitis is often more indolent with less severe symptoms (though may be just as dangerous).
- More atypical organisms such as fungal pathogens may also spread to the central nervous system (CNS), especially in immunocompromised individuals or individuals with abnormal exposures.

When Assessing a Patient with Possible Meningitis

- Perform a thorough history and general physical examination. Meningitis may present with multiple symptoms of infection including fever, chills, nausea, vomiting, or leukocytosis. CNS infections are often associated with seizures. Viral meningitis may be associated with more subtle changes including personality change, confusion, persistent headaches, and vague flu-like symptoms.
- Assess for signs of meningeal irritation including a Kernig test (extending the knee with passive hip flexion looking for sitting up or a verbal cry) and a Brudzinski sign (neck flexion resulting

in flexion of the hip). Assess for headaches, neck stiffness, photophobia, phonophobia, or vision changes (meningitis may cause increased intracranial pressure leading to papilledema).

- Perform a neurologic exam. Patients with signs of infection and changes in mental status or their neurologic exam (either or both) should be considered possible cases of meningitis.

- If meningitis is in the differential diagnosis, perform cerebrospinal fluid (CSF) analysis with a lumbar puncture. **You should have a very low threshold for performing a lumbar puncture.** Basically, if you think about it, you probably should do it.

- Prior to performing a lumbar puncture, make sure the patient has had a head CT. Lumbar punctures in the setting of lesions with mass effect may induce herniation. Nobody wants to be responsible for that! Do not perform a lumbar puncture if the patient is severely thrombocytopenic or has a coagulopathy.

- Like interviewing for residency, lumbar punctures can be intimidating, so be properly prepared. Don't rush and be cool and calm. Make sure the patient is properly positioned and thoroughly assess the anatomic landmarks. Set up the kit. Have an assistant.

- In the setting of suspected meningitis, attempt to obtain CSF prior to administering antibiotics. **Bacterial meningitis is yet another neurologic emergency. If there is any unavoidable delay in obtaining a diagnostic lumbar puncture, begin empiric treatment.**

- CSF should be sent for the following:
  - Cell count with differential in two tubes (the first and the last). This is important in case there is a high red blood cell count. Not that your lumbar punctures will ever be anything but champagne, of course. A rising red blood cell count raises the possibility of subarachnoid hemorrhage. See Table 22-1 for CSF analysis.
  - CSF protein, glucose, gram stain, bacterial cultures, and polymerase chain reactions (PCRs) for herpes simplex virus (HSV), varicella zoster virus (VZV), and cytomegalovirus (CMV).
  - If there is abnormal imaging, the patient is immunocompromised, or the patient has had usual exposures, consider CSF venereal disease research laboratory, cryptococcal antigen, fungal cultures, other viral PCRs, acid fast staining, and mycobacterial cultures.
  - An opening pressure can be very helpful in complex cases such as cryptococcal meningitis, so obtain it if possible. Remember, this is only accurate if the patient is lying on his/her side with the legs extended.

TABLE 22-1 CEREBROSPINAL FLUID ANALYSIS

Condition	Color	Pressure (mm H₂O)	Cells (#/mL)	Protein (mg/dL)	Glucose (mg/dL)
Normal	Clear	70-180	0-5 mononuclear	15-45 (may be higher with age)	45-80 (two-thirds of serum glucose)
Bacterial meningitis	Opalescent	Normal or ↑	>5 to many thousand PMNs	50-1500	0-45
Viral infection	Clear or opalescent	Normal or slightly ↑	>5-2000, mostly lymphocytes	20-200	Normal (may be slightly ↓)
Tuberculous meningitis	Clear or opalescent	Normal or ↑	>5-500 lymphocytes	45-500	10-45
Fungal meningitis	Clear or opalescent	Normal or ↑	>5-800 lymphocytes	Normal or ↑	Normal or ↓
Carcinomatous meningitis	Clear or opalescent	Normal or ↑	>5-1000, may include atypical cells	Up to 500	Normal or ↓
Subarachnoid hemorrhage	Bloody or xanthochromic	Normal or ↑	Many RBCs; ratio of WBC:RBC same as blood	Up to 2000	Normal

PMNs, polymorphonucleocytes; RBC, red blood cell; WBC, white blood cell.

- Treatment for meningitis typically should begin broadly with both bacterial and viral coverage. As with any suspected infection, obtain blood cultures prior to the initiation of antibiotics. Check your local protocol, but antibiotic coverage typically includes (at minimum) the following:
    - Ceftriaxone (2 g IV q12h) and vancomycin (dosed for weight and creatinine clearance)
    - Acyclovir (10 mg/kg of ideal body weight IV) until HSV, VZV, and CMV have been excluded
    - If the patient is at risk for listeria (elderly patients or immunocompromised patients), ampicillin (2 g IV q4h) should be added.

Obstetrics and Gynecology

Whitney Ross and Tammy Sonn

THE HISTORY AND PHYSICAL EXAMINATION

- **Perform a basic OB/GYN history and physical examination prior to calling a consult!** There are rare exceptions to this and "I don't want to" isn't one of them.
- **Gynecologic history**
  - Menstrual history
    - Last menstrual period (LMP)?
    - Age at menarche?
    - Age at menopause? Menopause = 1 full year without a menses. Any postmenopausal bleeding?
    - If a menstrual problem seems central to the chief complaint, ask about menstrual length, days between menses, amount of menstrual bleeding (e.g., number of pads used per day, how many hours it takes to saturate a pad), and the presence of dysmenorrhea. Normal menstrual flow is generally considered to be saturating through a pad or tampon every 2 hours or less on heavy days.
  - Pap history: Date of last pap test? Any history of abnormal paps?
  - Contraceptive history: Currently (or recently) using anything to prevent pregnancy?
  - Hormone use: Any history of exogenous hormone use (e.g., in perimenopausal women)?
  - Sexual history: Currently sexually active? History of any sexually transmitted infections (STIs)?
  - Gynecologic procedure history: Date and type of any gynecologic procedures/surgeries, for example, bilateral tubal ligation, diagnostic laparoscopy for endometriosis, unilateral or bilateral salpingo-oophorectomy, loop electrosurgical excision procedure?
  - **Clinical pearl**: Remember to include bowel and bladder function in any GYN history. Constipation and urinary tract infections are very common causes of pelvic complaints.

- **Obstetric history**
  - Ever been pregnant? How many times? Any complications? Any miscarriages?
  - If the patient is currently pregnant
    - Name of prenatal care provider/clinic? Estimated date of confinement or due date?
    - Any complications during this pregnancy?
    - If a pregnant patient is admitted to medical services, always give the OB/GYN consultation service a courtesy call even if the problem seems to be completely unrelated.
    - Any symptoms of vaginal bleeding, leakage of fluid, or decreased fetal movement? Any abdominal trauma? If yes, call OB urgently. Obviously.
- **Physical examination**: The physical examination may help you delineate between gynecologic versus nongynecologic causes of pelvic symptoms. Components may include the abdominal, vaginal speculum, and bimanual pelvic exams, in addition to a wet prep. What you are able to include will depend on your level of experience and access to materials.
- **Clinical pearl**: Pelvic exams are uncomfortable and no fun (for anyone). Make sure to differentiate between general discomfort and a Chandelier sign when palpating the cervix.
- **Examining the discharge**: The gonorrhea/chlamydia (GC/CT) test will take about 2 days. However, information can be gathered from point-of-care examination of any vaginal discharge you collected. On the wet prep, you might see white blood cells (associated with pelvic inflammatory disease [PID]), clue cells (associated with bacterial vaginosis), red blood cells (may be present with inflammation or active bleeding), or motile trichomonads. Do remember, not all moving cells are trichomonads. Any cell can move with the momentum of the wet prep fluid. Look for flagella and the characteristic corkscrew movement among stationary cells to distinguish. On the KOH prep, look for pseudohyphae (associated with candidiasis) or a positive whiff test (the presence of a fishy odor associated with bacterial vaginosis). A pH test can also be helpful—pH <4.5 may indicate normal vaginal flora or yeast, whereas a pH >4.5 is associated with bacterial vaginosis, trichomoniasis, gonorrhea, blood, or menopause.
- **Imaging**: Review any abdominopelvic MRI, CT, and ultrasounds that the patient already has. Bear in mind that a CT scan cannot always distinguish the characteristics of adnexal masses well; an

ultrasound is better. If further delineation of the pelvic organs is indicated, the OB/GYN consult team should be able to help guide you with which study to order and how it should be performed (sometimes OB/GYN will perform a pelvic ultrasound; at other institutions, it is performed by radiology).

VAGINAL DISCHARGE

Vaginitis

- The most common entities are bacterial vaginosis, vaginal candidiasis, and trichomoniasis.
- **Diagnosis**: The key symptoms, signs, and wet prep/KOH prep findings for the most common causes of infectious vaginitis are summarized in Table 23-1.
- **Treatment**: Listed here are the most common treatments for vaginitis. For additional treatment options, see www.cdc.gov.
  - **Vaginal candidiasis** (most commonly caused by *Candida albicans*)
    - **Fluconazole** 150 mg PO in a single dose (for severe infections or a compromised host, give a total of 2 to 3 doses to be taken q72h)
    - **Clotrimazole** 1% cream 1 applicator full intravaginally for 7 days (preferred option in pregnancy as opposed to oral option)
    - **Miconazole** 2% cream 1 applicator full intravaginally for 7 days (preferred option in pregnancy as opposed to oral option)
  - **Bacterial vaginosis**
    - **Metronidazole** 500 mg PO bid for 7 days
    - Metronidazole gel, 0.75%, 5 g intravaginally, once daily for 5 days
  - **Trichomoniasis** (because this is an STI, encourage the patient to have her partner treated)
    - **Metronidazole** 2 g PO in a single dose (preferred)
    - Metronidazole 500 mg PO bid for 7 days (alternative)

Cervicitis

- Cervicitis is most commonly caused by *Chlamydia trachomatis* and/or *Neisseria gonorrhoeae*. *Trichomonas vaginalis* is also associated with cervicitis.

TABLE 23-1   VAGINITIS

Condition	Symptoms	Exam Findings	pH	Wet Mount
Bacterial vaginosis	Increased discharge (thin, white) Increased odor	Thin, whitish-gray homogeneous discharge, sometimes frothy	>4.5	Clue cells (>20%) Amine odor after adding KOH (whiff test) Amsel criteria (need 3 of 4 for diagnosis): homogenous vaginal discharge, pH >4.5, clue cells (>20% of epithelial cells), +whiff test
Candidiasis	Increased discharge (white, thick) Pruritus Dysuria Burning	Thick, curd-like discharge Vaginal erythema	<4.5	Hyphae or spores Note: can be mixed infection with bacterial vaginosis, *Trichomonas vaginalis*, or both and have higher pH
Trichomoniasis	Increased discharge (yellow, frothy) Increased odor Pruritus Dysuria	Yellow, frothy discharge with or without vaginal or cervical erythema	>4.5	Motile trichomonads Increased white blood cells

Adapted from Eckert LO. Clinical practice: acute vulvovaginitis. N Engl J Med 2006;355:1244-52.

- **Diagnosis:** Suspect if yellow or green cervical discharge. The cervix may be inflamed (e.g., the "strawberry cervix" of trich). Perform a urine or endocervical GC/CT probe for definitive diagnosis. If cervical motion tenderness or pelvic pain is present, the diagnosis is PID, see the following section.
- **Treatment:** Adapted from the most recent Centers for Disease Control and Prevention (CDC) guidelines at www.cdc.gov (last accessed 1/1/2018). Encourage the patient to have her partner treated. Some states allow for expedited partner treatment, which authorizes you as the patient's physician to prescribe for the partner. Check your state's policies.
  - *N. gonorrhoeae*
    - Because of the rapidly developing antimicrobial resistance of *N. gonorrhoeae*, dual therapy should always be used and monotherapy is no longer acceptable.
    - **Ceftriaxone** 125 mg IM in a single dose PLUS **azithromycin** 1 g PO in a single dose (preferred)
    - **Cefixime** 400 mg PO in a single dose PLUS **azithromycin** 1 g PO in a single dose (second line, use if aforementioned is unavailable)
  - *C. trachomatis*
    - **Azithromycin** 1 g PO in a single dose (for easy dosing or if pregnant)
    - **Doxycycline** 100 mg PO bid for 7 days

Pelvic Inflammatory Disease

- PID is difficult to diagnose and can cause serious harm even when infection is mild, so the CDC advocates for providers to maintain a low threshold for treatment.
- **Clinical pearl:** <50% of women with PID will test positive for GC or CT.
- When no other source of illness is identified, empiric treatment of PID should be pursued in sexually active young women (and other women with risk factors for sexually transmitted diseases [STDs]) who have pelvic or lower abdominal pain and any one of the following:
  - Cervical motion tenderness OR
  - Uterine tenderness OR
  - Adnexal tenderness

- Mild to moderately severe PID can often be treated as an outpatient but requires inpatient treatment if patient is severely ill, is pregnant, has a tubo-ovarian abscess, is unable to tolerate an oral regimen, or is unable to follow up as an outpatient. If discharged from the emergency department or inpatient service, the patient should follow up within 72 hours of discharge. If no improvement, then inpatient management is indicated.

- Suboptimally treated PID can lead to infertility, chronic pelvic pain, sepsis, and even death. If treatment seems ineffective or the diagnosis is in question, please obtain an OB/GYN consultation.

- For treatment and diagnostic guidelines (cited earlier), see www. cdc.gov (last accessed 1/1/2018).

ECTOPIC PREGNANCY

- **Notify the OB/GYN team immediately if you suspect an ectopic pregnancy!**
- **History**
  - LMP
  - Missed menstrual period, date of first positive pregnancy test, abdominal pain, and/or vaginal spotting
  - Possible risk factors for ectopic pregnancy include prior ectopic pregnancy, history of tubal ligation or other tubal surgery, and history of prior gynecologic infection/PID.
- **Physical examination**
  - Vital signs: Include orthostatics (if patient is stable enough to stand up).
  - General: Note the degree of pallor, weakness, responsiveness, and pain.
  - Cardiovascular: Note the presence of tachycardia and quality of peripheral pulses.
  - Abdomen: May palpate the presence of a mass, rebound or guarding (signs of peritonitis), abdominal distension.
  - Pelvic exam: May or may not see bleeding at the cervical os, palpable cervical dilation, slightly enlarged uterus, and palpable adnexal mass.
- **Evaluation**
  - Complete blood count (CBC), type and screen, and urine human chorionic gonadotropin (hCG). If the urine is positive for hCG, obtain a quantitative serum β-hCG.

- Abdominal and pelvic ultrasound (including transvaginal) to determine location of pregnancy, gestational age, and fetal heart motion
- **Treatment**
  - IV access and fluid resuscitation (consider cross-matched blood if with any unstable vitals)
  - Medical (methotrexate) versus surgical management will be based on characteristics of the ectopic, stability of the patient, and patient preference. The OB/GYN consult team will determine the mode of treatment. I know, right?
  - **Clinical pearl**: Whenever vaginal bleeding or abdominal trauma occurs in a pregnant woman, make sure to obtain a type and screen. If Rh negative, anti-D immune globulin may be indicated to prevent fetal alloimmunization in future pregnancies.

ABNORMAL UTERINE BLEEDING

- Severity of bleeding will dictate the extent of your workup prior to calling a consult.
  - **If the patient has clinical symptoms of anemia and is actively bleeding heavily, please begin volume resuscitation and call an OB/GYN consult immediately!**
  - **If the patient has a known pregnancy or is of reproductive age with a positive urine pregnancy test, please call an OB/GYN consult immediately!**
- **History**
  - Menses information including LMP, frequency (days or weeks between bleeding), quantity (how many pad/tampon changes in 24 h or how many hours between changes), and duration of the bleeding
  - History of bleeding disorders
  - Medication usage (especially hormone therapy, contraception, or anticoagulants)
  - History of past gynecologic problems or a family history of gynecologic problems, including gynecologic cancer. **Suspect malignancy in any postmenopausal patient with vaginal bleeding.**
  - In the review of systems, address fevers, weight changes, general stress, chronic illness, bowel or bladder symptoms, or change in vaginal discharge.

- **Physical examination**
  - Abdominal, speculum, and pelvic exams should be performed to determine the source and extent of bleeding.
  - Rule out urologic and gastrointestinal sources of bleeding: spread the labia to inspect the urethra, send a macro/micro urinalysis (straight catheter specimen), and perform a digital rectal exam/guaiac (if rectal source suspected).
  - Vaginal bleeding may be coming from the uterus, the cervix itself, or the vaginal walls.
- **Evaluation**
  - CBC, type and screen, coagulation studies, serum hCG (if positive urine pregnancy test); consider thyroid-stimulation hormone and prolactin if with prolonged profile of abnormal uterine bleeding.
  - Imaging: abdominopelvic imaging (usually ultrasound) to characterize anatomic causes of bleeding (fibroids, polyps, ovarian masses, endometrial stripe thickness), and if pregnant, to determine the pregnancy status
  - Pathologic specimens
    - OB/GYN will perform pap and endometrial sampling if indicated. For more information on pap screening guidelines, see www.asccp.org/asccp-guidelines (last accessed 1/1/2018).
    - Postmenopausal women and women with chronic anovulation, obesity, or age greater than 45 years should have endometrial sampling. These women are at high risk for hyperplasia and malignancy.
- A simplified differential diagnosis is presented in Figure 23-1.
- Differential diagnosis by age group
  - 13 to 18 years: dysregulation of the hypothalamic-pituitary-ovarian axis (normal), pregnancy, hormonal contraceptive use, pelvic infection, coagulopathy, or tumors
  - 19 to 39 years: pregnancy, fibroids/polyps, anovulatory cycles, hormonal contraception, endometrial hyperplasia/cancer
  - 40 years to menopause: anovulatory bleeding (due to declining ovarian function), endometrial hyperplasia/cancer, endometrial atrophy if in menopause, fibroids/polyps, hormone therapy or hormonal contraception

Structural causes: PALM	Nonstructural causes: COEIN
Polyp	**C**oagulopathy
Adenomyosis	**O**vulatory dysfunction
Leiomyoma	**E**ndometrial
Malignancy	**I**atrogenic
	Not yet classified

Figure 23-1. Abnormal uterine bleeding differential diagnosis. (Adapted from Munro MG, Critchley HO, Broder MS, Fraser IS. FIGO classification system (PALM-COEIN) for causes of abnormal uterine bleeding in nongravid women of reproductive age. FIGO Working Group on Menstrual Disorders. *Int J Gynaecol Obstet* 2011;113:3-13, with permission.)

- **Treatment**
  - IV access, fluid resuscitation, transfusion as needed
  - Strict ins and outs, pad counts
  - Specific treatment will depend on etiology.

PELVIC MASS

- **Call an OB/GYN consult immediately if you suspect ovarian torsion! Ovarian torsion is a surgical emergency** and prompt surgical treatment could enable a young woman to keep her ovary.
- Ovarian torsion is clinically diagnosed. It may present with constant or intermittent severe abdominal pain, **a tender pelvic mass**, and low-grade temperatures. Pelvic ultrasound may demonstrate one enlarged ovary.
- **History**
  - Known history of fibroids or ovarian cysts in the past?
  - Pelvic mass growth—has there been any notable change in size?
  - Any weight changes, early satiety, abdominal girth increase, pain?
- **Physical examination**: Bimanual pelvic exam findings can help determine etiology—adnexal versus uterine origin. Abdominal exam may elicit a fluid wave.
- **Evaluation**
  - CBC and hCG (in reproductive age women). Specific tumor markers may be obtained in consultation with OB/GYN.
  - The OB/GYN consult team will help guide imaging. Transvaginal pelvic ultrasound will help to delineate the origin and internal features of the mass. If malignancy is suspected

or confirmed, further imaging (CT, MRI) may be indicated to determine the extent of disease. A barium enema or colonoscopy will help to exclude a gastrointestinal etiology.

- Differential diagnosis by age groups
  - 13 to 18 years: pregnancy, functional ovarian cysts (simple fluid-filled or simple blood-filled cysts), tubo-ovarian abscess, dermoid ovarian cysts, germ cell ovarian tumors, epithelial ovarian tumors, obstructing vaginal or uterine abnormalities
  - 19 years to menopause: pregnancy, functional ovarian cysts, tubo-ovarian abscess, hydrosalpinges, endometriomas, uterine fibroids, epithelial ovarian tumors
  - Postmenopausal: ovarian tumor (benign/malignant), fibroids, leiomyosarcoma, tubo-ovarian abscess, metastatic disease
- **Treatment**: varies greatly, depending on etiology

CONTRACEPTION

- Contraception is almost never an OB/GYN emergency.
- Medical eligibility for hormonal contraceptive options
  - Hormonal contraception carries varying degrees of risk as it relates to thrombotic risk, liver function in chronic disease, medication interactions, etc. Specific medical diagnoses may preclude the use of combined hormonal options or progestin only options.
  - We recommend using the US medical eligibility criteria for contraceptive use as a helpful guide, www.cdc.gov/reproductivehealth/contraception (last accessed 1/1/2018).
- Contraceptive options
  - **Long-acting reversible contraceptives** (LARC) are the most effective form of birth control. The major advantage is the lack of maintenance required by the patient to sustain its effectiveness. This should be the first recommendation given to women at higher risk of an unintended pregnancy (e.g., unable to remember daily pill taking). Obtain an OB/GYN consultation for any inpatient who you feel a LARC would be a good option.
    - Intrauterine device (IUD): The two main types are the hormonal (levonorgestrel releasing systems) versus nonhormonal (copper) options.
    - Implant: subdermal placement of etonogestrel in the upper arm

- **Combined oral contraceptive pills** are a very common form of contraception and cycle control. Typical dosing of the ethinylestradiol (EE) component will either be the ultralow dosing (10 µg EE), low dosing (20 µg EE), or mid dosing (30-35 µg EE). Several different progestin options exist with varying degrees of androgenic and antimineralocorticoid activity. If you have a patient who prefers pills and has side effects from her pills, consult an OB/GYN to further assist with decision-making regarding which EE dose and which progestin options would be best.
- Initiation of pill taking
  - **First day starts** mean the patient takes the first pill of a pack on the first day of her menses, assuming she has a regular menses. With compliant daily pill taking, she would not require 7 days of a backup method.
  - **Sunday starts** mean the patient takes the first pill of a pack on the first Sunday of her menses. She should not wait to take her first pill on a Sunday after her menses ends. This method has fallen out of favor. If this method is used, the patient should use a backup method for 7 days.
  - **Quick starting** means the patient starts the pill immediately, regardless of where she is in the menstrual cycle (after confirmation of a negative pregnancy test). This has been shown to improve adherence in adolescents. Backup contraception for the first 7 days is required prior to relying on the pill.
- **Transdermal patches** are a combination option that delivers a low dose of EE (20 µg) and progestin hormone daily. This patch is applied 1× per week for 3 weeks with 1 patch-free week when the patient will experience a withdrawal menses. Typical locations for the patch include lower abdomen, upper buttocks, upper outer arm, and upper torso. Initiation of patch usage follows the same rules as pill taking.
- **Vaginal rings** are a combination option, which releases a low dose of EE (15 µg) and progestin hormone daily. This flexible ring is placed in the vaginal canal and left in place for 3 weeks. The ring is removed at the start of the 4th week and menses typically occurs. If the ring is expulsed for more than 3 hours, replace the ring after simple washing and use backup contraception for 7 days. If the ring was expulsed for less than 3 hours, wash and replace with no need for backup contraception. Initiation of ring usage follows the same rules as pill taking.

- **Depo-Provera** injections are a progestin only injectable option given every 3 months. This can be initiated on any day with the same initiation rules as pill taking. Patients must return to the office for injection visits. Since this is a progestin only option, more patients may be able to safely have this as a contraceptive option compared with combination hormonal options.
- **Progestin only pills** provide a pill version progestin only option. This pill pack has an active daily pill with no placebo pills. The patient must feel she can be compliant with daily pill taking. The most effective method is taking the tablet at the same time daily. If pill is more than 3 hours late, backup contraception is needed and the patient should read package insert guidelines to determine next best steps. Initiation of this pill follows the same rules as combination pills.
- See Table 23-2 for details comparing the unintended pregnancy rates among different options.
- Emergency contraceptive options: Assist in preventing pregnancy after an unprotected sexual intercourse encounter (no contraception, condom breaking, inconsistent use of pill/patch/ring). Table 23-3 lists the available methods of emergency contraception.

TABLE 23-2	CONTRACEPTIVE OPTIONS: 1ST YEAR UNINTENDED PREGNANCY RATES	
Contraceptive Method	**Typical Use (%)**	**Perfect Use (%)**
Copper intrauterine device	0.8	0.6
Levonorgestrel intrauterine device	0.2	0.2
Etonogestrel implant	0.05	0.05
Combined pill/progestin-only pill	9	0.3
Female sterilization	0.5	0.5
Male sterilization	0.15	0.1

Adapted from Trussell J. Contraceptive failure in the United States. Contraception *2011;83:397-404.*

TABLE 23-3	METHODS OF EMERGENCY CONTRACEPTION	

Method	Number of Days After Unprotected Sexual Intercourse	Prescription Required? (Y/N)
Progestin only		
1.5 mg levonorgestrel × 1	Up to 3 d	No
0.75 mg levonorgestrel q12h × 2	Up to 3 d	No
Combined progestin-estrogen pills (100 µg EE + 0.5 mg levonorgestrel q12h × 2)	Up to 5 d	Yes
Copper IUD	Up to 5 d	Yes (with office visit for insertion)
Selective progesterone receptor modulator (ulipristal acetate 30 mg × 1)	Up to 5 d	Yes

IUD, intrauterine device.

Ophthalmology

Iris Lee, Han Li, and Morton Smith

RSVP

- Consider calling ophthalmology for any of these signs/symptoms, especially if there are more than one.
  - Redness: By itself, this is the least specific sign for pathology. Causes of red eye can range from more benign causes such as allergy and dry eye to endophthalmitis and uveitis.
  - Sensitivity to light: Ask the patient, does the light hurt your eyes?
  - Vision change: Clarify whether there is blurriness, actual vision loss, double vision, or positive phenomenon such as flashes or floaters.
  - Pain: Try to clarify whether the pain is anterior (often described as burning, scratching, sand, twigs, or "something IN my eye," associated with dry eye, corneal abrasion, etc.) or posterior (throbbing, aching, or boring, associated with uveitis, endophthalmitis, etc.).
- **Clinical pearl**: Redness, sensitivity to light, blurry vision, and anterior eye pain can be seen with dry eye. Most patients who are intubated or sedated get dry eye—they should be on lacrilube.

COMMON DROPS THAT THE PATIENT MAY BE TAKING

- **Dilating (red)**: phenylephrine, tropicamide, cyclopentolate, atropine
- **Antibiotics (tan)**: ofloxacin (Ocuflox), moxifloxacin (Vigamox)
- **Steroid (white/pink)**: loteprednol (Lotemax), prednisolone (Pred Forte), difluprednate (Durezol)
- **Allergy**: ketotifen (Zaditor), olopatadine (Patanol)
- **Glaucoma**: latanoprost (Xalatan), travoprost (Travatan), brimonidine (Alphagan), brimonidine and timolol (Combigan), brinzolamide (Azopt), timolol (Timoptic)
- **Anesthetic**: proparacaine

THE OPHTHALMOLOGIC HISTORY AND EXAMINATION

- Basic ophthalmic **history**
  - Vision: acute or chronic, bilateral or unilateral, central or peripheral, painful or painless, constant or intermittent
  - Prior ophthalmic history: known ophthalmic conditions, prior eye surgery or trauma, contact lens/eye medication use, and relevant medical/family history
- Basic ophthalmic **physical examination**
  - **Vision: Best corrected** visual acuity (**extremely important**). Test each eye **individually** with **correction** (glasses, contacts) and **good lighting.** If no vision chart is available, have the patient attempt to read your name badge or any other printed materials in his/her room. If the patient is unable to read the top line of the chart or newspaper headlines, evaluate by asking the patient to count fingers, or detect hand motions or the presence of light.
  - **Pupils:** Are the pupils/iris equally clear through the cornea? Are they round and equal in size? Do they react to light? Is there an afferent pupillary defect with the swinging flashlight test?
  - **Motility and alignment**: Are the eyes aligned when the patient is looking straight ahead (primary gaze)? Is motility full? Is there nystagmus?
  - **Visual field:** Test **each** individual eye, usually performed by counting fingers in the peripheral vision (1, 2, and 5 are easy to distinguish).
  - **External exam:** Are the eyes proptotic? Is eyelid position normal? Is the eye red?
  - **Fundus exam:** Determine whether there is a red reflex (can be unequal if there are opacities in the vitreous such as blood or infection) by looking at the patient through the ophthalmoscope from 1 to 2 feet away. Focus on optic nerve pathology ("CBC" explained in the following text). Anything else on the exam is a bonus (retinal hemorrhage, retinal detachment). It is often helpful to communicate the level of confidence of your fundus exam to the consultant. And honestly, for many of us...
  - **Clinical pearl:** Follow **CBC** to remember the optic nerve exam. Color should be pink (white implies prior nerve damage). Border should be crisp (if blurred or feathery think elevated intracranial pressure). Cup should be <50% (if greater than this, think glaucoma).

THE RED EYE

See Figure 24-1.

Conjunctivitis

- **History**: recent upper respiratory tract infection (URI)/sick contacts, exposures, allergies, or history of allergic conjunctivitis
- **Clinical presentation/physical examination**
  - Viral: unilateral red eye (can be bilateral if spread to the other eye), possible associated URI symptoms, mild itching, morning crusting or watery discharge, follicles
  - Allergic: bilateral itching, mild redness, watery discharge, lid swelling, chemosis (edema of the conjunctiva), papillae
  - Bacterial: **acute purulent discharge**, eyelid edema, decreased vision
- **Evaluation**: For possible bacterial conjunctivitis, perform Gram stain and culture of discharge.
- **Treatment**
  - Viral: No specific medical treatment necessary, self-limited illness. **Hand hygiene** (most important). Wash towels and pillowcases. Use separate towels. Symptomatic treatment with cool compresses or artificial tears. No contact lens use until asymptomatic for at least 7 days.

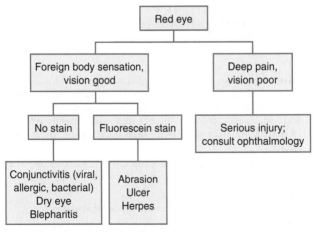

Figure 24-1. Algorithm for the red eye.

- Allergic: Eliminate inciting agent. Cool compresses and artificial tears. Oral antihistamines. Antihistamine drops per ophthalmology.
- Bacterial: Systemic treatment for gonorrhea and chlamydia if clinical concern for sexually stransmitted infections (STIs) or proven with ocular cultures. Treat sexual partners. Ointment and antibiotic drops per ophthalmology.
- **Clinical pearls**
  - Allergic and viral conjunctivitis should not have severely decreased vision or pain.
  - Always wear gloves if you suspect viral conjunctivitis.
  - Use of eye drops with vasoconstrictors (e.g., Visine, Clear eyes) can cause rebound redness. Avoid empiric treatment with these medications.

Scleritis

- **History:** previous episodes, symptoms suggestive of associated systemic disease, **deep/boring pain**, vision loss
- **Physical examination**
  - Redness of the eye (can be diffuse or sectoral)
  - Pain on palpation of the eye (over the eyelid) or with eye movement
  - Inflamed scleral vessels cannot be moved with a cotton-tipped applicator.
  - May see thinning of the sclera (blue).
- **Treatment:** First line is NSAIDS, per ophthalmology consultation. Steroids if NSAID failure.

Uveitis

- **History:** previous episodes, symptoms suggestive of associated systemic disease (e.g., autoimmune, Lyme, tuberculosis, syphilis, sarcoid), recent cataract surgery or trauma, medications (e.g., rifabutin, cidofovir, sulfonamides, pamidronate, systemic moxifloxacin), **light sensitivity, deep/boring pain**, vision loss/floaters
- **Physical examination:** cell/flare, hypopyon (e.g., layer of pus at the bottom of the anterior chamber), abnormally shaped pupil
- **Treatment**
  - Cycloplegia and topical steroids, per ophthalmology
  - Workup and treatment of underlying systemic disease

INFECTION

Endophthalmitis

- **Endophthalmitis is an ocular emergency of the highest degree. Call a consult immediately!** Time is vision.
- **History**: history of recent ocular surgery (cataract, glaucoma), bloodstream infection, or trauma; unilateral **painful eye; decreased vision** (often severe)
- **Physical examination**: red eye, hypopyon, poor red reflex or view to the back of the eye
- **Treatment**
  - Emergent ophthalmologic evaluation, keep the patient NPO.
  - May need culture and intravitreal antibiotics.

Herpes/Varicella Zoster Virus

- **History**: Immunocompromised/HIV, preceding vesicular rashes; blurred vision, eye pain, red eye; may have skin rash and discomfort.
- **Physical examination**: Skin vesicles in dermatomal distribution respecting the midline (Hutchinson sign for varicella zoster—the eye is more likely involved if rash involves the tip of the nose), conjunctivitis, uveitis, scleritis, cranial nerve palsy
- **Treatment**
  - If younger than 40 years, evaluate for immunosuppression.
  - Oral antivirals
  - Antibiotic ointments and drops per ophthalmology

INJURY

Trauma With Possible Ruptured Globe

- Put that stick down! You'll put someone's eye out!
- **Ocular emergency, call for a consultation immediately!**
- **History**: history of events preceding trauma, specific chemicals or items involved, any history of possible foreign body (e.g., hammering on metal), anything else that is currently going on medically; pain, decreased vision
- **Physical examination** findings suggestive of a ruptured globe: Severely decreased vision (count fingers or worse), 360° subconjunctival hemorrhage, full-thickness corneal or scleral laceration, peaked or irregular pupil, shallow anterior chamber, hyphema (i.e., blood in the anterior chamber), exposed intraocular contents. Now doesn't that sound fun?

- **Treatment**
  - Place a shield over the involved eye. **Do not press on the eye or touch ocular contents.** Little chance of that.
  - Keep the patient NPO (determine last meal) and on bed rest.
  - IV antibiotics: moxifloxacin IV (per ophthalmology)
  - Tetanus toxoid as needed
  - Antiemetic as needed to prevent Valsalva, pain control
  - CT of the orbits (axial and coronal)
  - Surgical repair

Chemical Burn

- Basically, alkali is worse than acid. Get it? Basically?
- **Ocular urgency! Start irrigation with sterile solution before calling ophthalmology immediately.**
- **History:** history of the event, specific chemicals and amounts involved, time/duration of contact, duration of irrigation at scene; possible pain, blurry vision, foreign body sensation, tearing, photophobia
- **Physical examination**
  - Mild to moderate injury: corneal epithelial defects, red eye, mild chemosis, eyelid edema, first- or second-degree periocular skin burns
  - Moderate to severe: pronounced chemosis, perilimbal (junction of cornea and sclera) blanching, corneal edema or opacification, anterior chamber reaction, increased intraocular pressure, second- or third-degree burns
- Immediate **treatment** (prior to contacting consult service)
  - **Irrigate, irrigate, irrigate,** with any available sterile solution (e.g., 0.9% saline, 0.45% saline, or lactated Ringer's), and keep irrigating until you talk with the consultant.
  - **Do not use acid or alkali to neutralize.** Yeah, that just sounds wrong.
  - Check pH 5 minutes after irrigation; continue irrigation until pH is neutral (i.e., pH 7).

Corneal Ulcer

- **This is an ocular urgency rather than an emergency.**
- **History:** previous ulcers or herpetic infections, history leading up to event (recent trauma, especially with vegetable matter, or

sleeping or swimming in contact lenses), topical anesthetic use; pain, photophobia, red eye, decreased vision, with or without discharge

- **Physical examination**: focal corneal opacity and overlying epithelial defect (abrasion), anterior chamber reaction with or without hypopyon, eyelid edema, lagophthalmos (incomplete eyelid closure)
- **Evaluation**: Routine cultures of corneal scrapings (done by ophthalmologist) include Gram stain, KOH prep, and fungal culture.
- **Treatment**
  - Pain control
  - Cycloplegia, topical antibiotic treatment per ophthalmology. Antibiotic selection depends on size and location of ulcer and association with contact lens use; usually a fluoroquinolone such as levofloxacin or moxifloxacin is first line (ciprofloxacin drops can cause additional irritation).
  - No contact lens wear
- **Clinical pearl**: Contact lens wearers are at much higher risk. Etiology can be bacterial, fungal, HSV, and *Acanthamoeba* spp. Patients who cannot close their eyes fully are at increased risk for exposure keratopathy and corneal ulcers (e.g., ICU patients).

Corneal Abrasion or Foreign Body

- **History**: occurrences leading up to event, immediate onset after procedure during which patient is sedated, occupational history (i.e., grinding, drilling, trauma), **contact lens use**, type of foreign body, prior abrasion/erosion; acute pain, tearing, photophobia, blurry vision, foreign body sensation.
- **Evaluation**
  - Look for associated corneal ulcers (white opacity seen before fluorescein instilled).
  - Examine with fluorescein to detect epithelial defect (green fluorescent spot under cobalt blue light).
  - Look for foreign body or rust ring.
  - Measure and record dimension of defect.
  - Evert eyelids to look for hidden foreign bodies.
- **Treatment**
  - **Remove foreign body** (preferably by an ophthalmologist).
  - Noncontact lens wearers: Treat with bacitracin/polymyxin or erythromycin ointment q2-4h (ointment preferred to drops for symptomatic relief).

- Contact lens wearers: Must have pseudomonal coverage (i.e., ofloxacin). No contact lens use until cleared by an ophthalmologist.
- Cycloplegia
- Follow up the next day with an ophthalmologist and follow up as needed thereafter.
- **Clinical pearl**: If a patient has eye pain, redness, or foreign body sensation immediately after returning from a procedure requiring sedation, it is likely a postoperative corneal abrasion. This can be managed conservatively by the primary team with a trial of erythromycin ointment q4 hours. However, if the history is suggestive of direct trauma or there is any chance of penetrating injury, call a consult immediately.

PAINLESS ACUTE VISION LOSS

Central Retinal Artery Occlusion

- Yet another major big deal! Essentially a stroke of the eye.
- **History: painless, unilateral**, acute loss of vision; history of amaurosis fugax (i.e., painless, temporary, monocular vision loss). Ask about symptoms of giant cell arteritis (GCA).
- **Physical examination**: pale retina with a so-called cherry red spot at the fovea, afferent pupillary defect, narrowed arterioles, occasionally arteriolar emboli/plaque visible (Hollenhorst plaque), vision usually counting fingers or worse
- **Evaluation**: HbA1c, complete blood count, coagulation tests, blood pressure, carotid duplex, echocardiogram. Check erythrocyte sedimentation rate/C-reactive protein in patients with high suspicion of GCA. In younger patients, consider further labs depending on review of systems (e.g., antinuclear antibody, rheumatoid factor, syphilis serology, serum protein electrophoresis, sickle cell test, and hypercoagulable labs).
- **Treatment**
  - Call an ophthalmologist! Permanent visual loss likely after 90 to 120 minutes. However, there are no reliable treatments to reverse central retinal artery occlusion.
  - Ocular massage (anecdotal): Have patient close eyes, apply pressure to the globe for 5 to 15 seconds, and then release. Repeat several times.
- **Clinical pearl**: Ask about symptoms of GCA (fever, weight loss, unilateral **headache**, polymyalgia rheumatic, **jaw claudication**, scalp tenderness) in all patients >50 years of age.

Retinal Detachment

- **An ocular urgency**
- **History**: preceding trauma or surgery, ocular history, oncologic history (melanoma, hematologic), history of proliferative diabetic retinopathy; painless unilateral **decreased vision with associated flashes and floaters** (often hundreds or thousands in number), curtain or veil across vision, visual field defect
- **Physical examination**: Usually no afferent pupillary defect unless a large retinal detachment. Fundus exam reveals a white, billowing, or wrinkled retina; may be able to see difference in red reflex depending on the size of the detachment.
- **Evaluation**: slit-lamp exam and dilated fundus exam
- **Treatment**: Call ophthalmology because you totally don't know what you're doing.

PAINFUL ACUTE VISION LOSS

Acute Angle-Closure Glaucoma

- **Ocular emergency, call a consult immediately!**
- **History**: current meds (e.g., antihistamines, mydriatics) including ocular medications, family history of angle closure, recent eye surgery/laser, cardiovascular/pulmonary status, electrolyte/renal status; **severe pain**, blurry vision, colored halos around lights, frontal headache, **nausea/vomiting**
- **Physical examination**: conjunctival injection; **fixed, mid-dilated pupil**; shallow anterior chamber; **acutely elevated intraocular pressure, hazy cornea**
- **Evaluation**: slit-lamp exam; measure intraocular pressure.
- **Treatment**
  - Pain and nausea control as needed.
  - Medical treatment involves ophthalmic drops and systemic medications to decrease intraocular pressure and medications to manage associated inflammation—consult ophthalmology first.
  - Laser treatment. No, you totally don't know how to do that.
- **Clinical pearl**: Cardiovascular and pulmonary status can be affected by glaucoma drops. Electrolyte/renal status should be known before administering acetazolamide.

DOUBLE VISION

* **Binocular diplopia can be a neurologic and/or ophthalmologic emergency (but not always).**
* It is defined as double vision resulting from the two eyes not being aligned.
* Test for this by covering each of the eyes individually and asking if the double vision resolves. **If the double vision is present with both eyes open, but then goes away when covering each eye separately, then the patient has binocular diplopia.**
* **History**
  * Stroke risk factors, neurologic history (e.g., myasthenia gravis, multiple sclerosis), intracranial process (e.g., malignancy), head trauma, intraorbital process (e.g., cellulitis, thyroid eye disease, malignancy), sedating medications
  * The patient presents with intermittent or constant diplopia, with vertical, horizontal, or oblique double images.
  * May be associated with neurologic symptoms, e.g., weakness, numbness, vertigo, headache.
  * **If the diplopia is new and constant, strongly consider neurologic causes** (e.g., cranial nerve palsies including 3rd, 4th, or 6th).
* **Physical examination**: Misaligned eyes in the primary position or in certain directions of gaze. Check for ptosis, anisocoria, and exophthalmos.
* **Treatment**: Consider noncontrast head CT if there is concern for intracranial hemorrhage. Otherwise, may need to consider orbital CT or brain MRI with orbital cuts with ophthalmology and/or neurology guidance.

Orthopedic Surgery

Zachary Meyer, Kimberly Bartosiak, and Martin Boyer

PRIOR TO CALLING THE CONSULT

- A thorough **physical examination** of the patient should be made **before** calling an orthopedic consult. This should include neurovascular exam (e.g., pulses, sensation, and motor function) of the involved extremity. All wounds should also be examined. Skipping this step will definitely make you look dumb. It would sort of be like calling a cardiology consult prior to listening to the patient's heart. Poor form dude.
- **Radiographs** of the affected joint/bone should also be obtained before calling an ortho consult. Resist the urge to call a consult before obtaining radiographs (see the following text for exceptions). This will sometimes be very difficult, but you must try. Usually two views, an anteroposterior (AP) and a lateral view, of the affected area are sufficient. Special cases are listed.
  - **Shoulder/proximal humerus**: AP, true AP, axillary, scapular lateral (or Y) views. The axillary view is especially important. This can be hard for the radiology technician to perform when the patient has a painful shoulder, but this view is essential to determine that the shoulder is not dislocated.
  - **Hip fractures** (femoral neck/intertrochanteric fractures): AP hip, cross-table lateral (not a frog leg lateral), AP ortho pelvis (an AP pelvis centered on the inferior half of the pelvis)
  - **Pelvis/acetabular fractures**: AP ortho pelvis, Judet (oblique) views, inlet/outlet views
  - **Ankle**: AP, lateral, mortise views
  - **Foot**: AP, lateral, medial oblique views; and a Harris heel (axial) view if a calcaneus fracture is suspected
  - Consultation with the orthopedic service is preferred, prior to obtaining a CT, MRI, or bone scan, and plain films should always be obtained prior to ordering more advanced imaging.
- For fractures, acute dislocations, suspected compartment syndrome, joint sepsis, cauda equina syndrome, or diabetic infections; make patients NPO and discontinue all anticoagulants.

- If not already done, order typical preoperative labs as indicated: complete blood count (CBC), basic or complete metabolic panel (BMP or CMP), prothrombin time/international normalized ratio, partial thromboplastin time, and type and screen. If infection is suspected, include an erythrocyte sedimentation rate (ESR) and C-reactive protein (CRP). If the patient is febrile, obtain blood cultures.
- Certain orthopedic issues are better managed in an outpatient setting. Examples include chronic pain in the spine or extremity, rotator cuff tears, ankle sprains, patients requesting joint injections. For these types of problems, consider having the patient follow-up with an orthopedist once he/she is discharged from the hospital, rather than calling an inpatient orthopedic consult.
- Consider medical or general surgical causes of orthopedic symptoms, such as cholecystitis causing right shoulder pain, myocardial ischemia causing left shoulder pain, and inguinal hernia causing hip pain.
- If an orthopedist has operated on the patient within the past several months, even for an unrelated problem, consider a courtesy call to alert the orthopedist that the patient has been admitted. Any unexpected hospital admissions may affect the patient's post-op rehab course.

FRACTURES

- **History**: mechanism of injury and preinjury level of activity (e.g., does the patient walk, does he/she use a walker, is he/she wheelchair bound, what kind of work does he/she do?)
- **Physical examination**: Complete distal neurologic and vascular exam. Examine joints proximal and distal to the injury. Carefully examine all extremities to rule out other injuries. Take down splints/dressings to perform exams, unless the fracture has been reduced by another physician or outside hospital prior to your exam. Err on the side of taking down the dressing, as open fractures have been missed by referring emergency departments. Oops!
- **Describing fractures**: For bonus points, attempt to delineate the following prior to calling a consult. It is okay if your description is woefully incorrect. Sometimes, even the ortho team isn't sure how to describe a fracture but they will nevertheless find your attempt either very amusing and charmingly naïve or very impressive. It's a win-win.
  - Bone: Although patients may disagree, the tibula or fibula is not a bone.
  - Fracture pattern: transverse, oblique, spiral

- Displacement: How far are the fragments away from each other? Which direction, anterior, posterior, medial, or lateral?
- Angulation: By how many degrees do the fragments relate to each other?
- Shortening: How much do the fragments overlap?
- Comminution: Is it a clean break or are there multiple small fragments about the fracture site?
- Open versus closed: Any break in the skin in the vicinity of a fracture must be considered an open fracture until proven otherwise with a careful examination of the wound. Ouch!
- Always attempt to review the radiographs and not just the radiology reads. Orthopedic surgery residents have excellent reading skills.
- **Initial management**
  - Keep patients NPO until evaluated by the ortho team.
  - Closed fractures are treated on an individual basis and on the basis of particular bone involvement and amount of displacement.
  - **Open fractures require urgent or emergent operative debridement and fixation.** Um, excuse me doctor. That's just my bone sticking out. I'll be fine.
    - **Open fractures and fractures with associated neurovascular compromise** are emergencies. Order radiographs and basic pre-op labs, make the patient NPO, discontinue any anticoagulants, and **call a consult immediately!** Any open wound in the same limb segment as a fracture means that the fracture is open unless proven otherwise by the orthopedic resident.
    - **Clinical pearl: If you see a poke hole in the skin near a fracture that will not stop oozing, the fracture is open!**
    - Open fractures require a tetanus booster and antibiotics, usually cefazolin with or without gentamicin depending on the size and contamination of the wound. Orthopedic surgery residents do not believe in the notion of too much cefazolin; however, in general, 1 to 2 g is sufficient. If there is fecal or barnyard contamination of the wound, consider anaerobic coverage (metronidazole or clindamycin) as well. Um, gross!
    - Open fractures often attract a crowd, but once they have been evaluated by critical personnel, it is best for the patient to keep the wound covered with a dressing.

SEPTIC JOINT

- **This is an emergency!** Call for an ortho consultation immediately after complete examination, radiographs, and labs are obtained. Make the patient NPO and discontinue any anticoagulants.
- **History:** warmth, painful range of motion, tenderness, fever, inability to ambulate/use extremity
- **Physical examination:** neurovascular exam (e.g., pulses, sensation, motor), effusion/fluctuance, erythema, warmth, considerable pain with passive range of motion
- **Evaluation:** Plain radiographs, CBC, BMP, ESR, CRP, and blood cultures (if febrile). The diagnosis is by arthrocentesis. Aspiration may be done by the primary physician or an orthopedic consultant. Do not aspirate a joint through cellulitis if at all possible. Synovial fluid should be sent for stat Gram stain, cell count, crystals, and cultures (aerobic and anaerobic). Antibiotics should not be administered until a joint aspirate is obtained.
- **Diagnosis**
  - Septic arthritis is diagnosed with a synovial fluid leukocyte count generally >50,000/mm^3, a positive Gram stain, or a positive culture result.
  - An inflammatory/autoimmune arthropathy typically has a synovial fluid leukocyte count of 10,000 to 50,000/mm^3, with positive crystals (for gout or calcium pyrophosphate deposition disease) and negative Gram stain and culture results.
  - Prosthetic joint infections may present differently and have a different set of diagnostic criteria. It is preferable to involve orthopedics prior to obtaining an aspiration.
- **Treatment**
  - Operative drainage: *Neisseria* spp. are exceptions to this rule, as they are highly responsive to antibiotic therapy; operative debridement is not necessary. A privately taken history may be of great importance in these cases.
  - Appropriate intravenous antibiotics as determined by cultures. The course of antibiotics is typically 6 weeks. Consider an infectious disease consultation and long-term venous access if IV antibiotics are needed.
- **Clinical pearls:** *Staphylococcus aureus* is the most common organism in septic arthritis. *Neisseria gonorrhoeae* is also prevalent in sexually active adolescents and adults. *Salmonella* is something to consider in patients with sickle cell, although *S. aureus* is still the most common organism in this patient population.

COMPARTMENT SYNDROME

- **Compartment syndrome is an emergency! Call a consult imme-diately**, after complete examination and radiographs. Make the patient NPO and discontinue any anticoagulants.

- Compartment syndromes are caused by **elevated hydrostatic pressure within a fixed osteofascial space**, leading to tissue ischemia as compartment pressure exceeds capillary pressure (i.e., the pressure in the compartment prevents blood flow out of and into the affected area). Elevated hydrostatic pressure commonly occurs from bleeding or swelling from within the compartment or from persistently elevated externally applied pressure.

- The most specific signs and symptoms of compartment syndrome are pain out of proportion to injury, pain with passive stretch of the muscles in the involved compartment, and hard tense compartments. Paresthesias, pallor, pulselessness, and paralysis may or may not be present (all are more indicative of arterial insufficiency). All external circumferential dressings should be removed before examining a patient for compartment syndrome.

- **History**: A typical history may include trauma (fracture or muscle contusion), ischemia (vascular injury, extended compression), venous obstruction, massive inflammation from snake or insect bites, bleeding into the compartment (consider in anticoagulated patients, infiltration of fluid into a compartment (paint gun injuries, IV infiltration), and tight circumferential dressings (Um, isn't that called a tourniquet?).

- **Physical examination**: Directly palpate the concerning area to determine tightness/turgor of compartments. Compare with the contralateral side. Passively range the muscles that traverse the compartment (i.e., in the forearm, passively flex and extend the fingers). Check for pulses, sensation, and motor function. Continue to monitor the patient with serial exams and elevate the concerning extremity to the level of the heart.

- When clinical signs are equivocal or when the patient is obtunded or not cooperative with the exam, compartment pressures may be measured by an orthopedic consultant. Compartment pressures >30 mm Hg (or a diastolic blood pressure to compartment pressure difference <30 mm Hg in hypotensive patients) are diagnostic of compartment syndrome. In general compartment syndrome is a clinical diagnosis and compartment pressure measurements are obtained in only a minority of cases.

- **Treatment**: Make patient NPO immediately upon suspicion of diagnosis. Obtain plain radiographs and any indicated pre-op labs. If compartment syndrome is confirmed, the orthopedics team will proceed with **emergent fasciotomy.**
- **Clinical pearls**: Remember that rhabdomyolysis can occur with compartment syndrome from muscle necrosis. Administer IV fluids, follow up urine output, creatinine, and creatine kinase.

ACUTE CAUDA EQUINA SYNDROME

- **This is an emergency, call a consult immediately** after examination and radiographs. Again, make the patient NPO and discontinue any anticoagulants.
- Cauda equina syndrome is caused by a lesion in the spinal canal located in the lumbar spine, between the conus medullaris and the lumbosacral nerve roots, resulting in urinary retention, bowel incontinence, saddle anesthesia, severe lower extremity neurologic deficit, and anal sphincter laxity.
- **History**: Suspect in a patient with low back pain and the previously mentioned signs and symptoms. It is helpful to clarify if they have true incontinence or are having too much pain to make it to the restroom.
- **Physical examination**: A complete lower extremity neurologic exam should be performed including lower extremity strength, sensation, and reflexes. A rectal exam must be performed to assess both rectal tone and perianal sensation. Remember that the cauda equina functions as the peripheral nervous system. Therefore, in a complete cauda equina injury, all peripheral nerves to the bowel, bladder, perianal area, and lower extremities will be lost, resulting in absent lower extremity tendon, bulbo-cavernosus, anal reflexes. (My goodness!) Nerve root tension signs such as pain on straight leg raise are likely to be present as well. On occasion, pain may radiate down the leg that is not being flexed (crossover pain) in addition to radiating down the leg being flexed.
- **Evaluation**: Stat AP and lateral views of the lumbar spine and a stat MRI of the lumbar spine without contrast.
- **Treatment**: Keep patient NPO, obtain necessary pre-op blood work, and discontinue anticoagulants. If cauda equine syndrome is confirmed, the orthopedic spine team will proceed with emergent operative decompression.

DIABETIC FOOT ULCER/INFECTIONS

- The acuity of these infections is dictated by the patient's systemic symptoms. If the patient is febrile and/or hemodynamically unstable, call a consult immediately.

- Diabetic ulcerations occur after patients lose the protective sensation in their feet. Patients may present with an advanced infection because of lack of pain.

- **History**: recent glycemic control (have insulin requirements been increasing in order to maintain the same level of plasma glucose?), prior amputations or debridements, history of optic or renal dysfunction, or cardiac disease

- **Physical examination**: Obtain a thorough neurovascular exam including pulses, sensation, and motor function. Examine all wounds taking note of depth, purulence, necrotic tissue, exposed bone, and proximal extension. If peripheral pulses are absent or diminished, perform an ankle brachial index and consider vascular surgery consultation (see "Ischemic Ulcer of the Lower Extremity" section in Chapter 28, General Surgery).

- **Evaluation**: CBC, BMP, coagulation panel, ESR, and CRP. Obtain AP, lateral, and oblique views of the ankle and foot. Do not obtain an MRI prior to an orthopedic consultation.

- **Treatment**: Surgical management will vary on the basis of the wound and can range from bedside debridement to limb amputation. Antimicrobial therapy should be based upon tissue or bone culture results when possible but broad-spectrum agents (e.g., piperacillin/tazobactam or meropenem with or without vancomycin) should be started promptly for signs of hemodynamic compromise. Consider an infectious diseases consultation, as well as placement of a long-term venous access device if an extended course of IV antibiotics is anticipated.

ONCOLOGICAL ISSUES

- The cancers that most commonly metastasize to the bone are breast, prostate, lung, thyroid, and renal cell carcinoma. Less common cancers are multiple myeloma, leukemia, lymphoma, and melanoma.

- **Any oncology patient with pain in an extremity or in the spine may have a bony metastasis and an impending fracture.** The appropriate radiographs should be obtained, and an orthopedic consult should be called if a lesion is visualized. Impending fractures are important to recognize and treat early because once the bone is fractured, fixation can become much more difficult.

- Oncology patients with spinal metastases resulting in neurologic compromise may do better with surgical decompression than with radiation alone. An orthopedic consult should be called for these patients too.

MANAGEMENT OF POSTOPERATIVE ORTHOPEDIC PATIENTS

- Orthopedic patients are frequently admitted to a general medicine service (often to the dismay of said service) postoperatively for significant medical comorbidities or unexpected medical complications.
- Orthopedic procedures can result in significant blood loss, so labs should be carefully followed up in the 48 hours following any surgery. Special attention should be given to the hematocrit, coagulation studies, and urine output. It is not unusual for the patient's hematocrit to decrease over the 48 hours following a large orthopedic procedure. Therapeutic anticoagulation should be started without discussing it with the orthopedic team.
- For all orthopedic patients, and especially patients with hip or pelvic pathology, there is a particularly high risk of deep venous thrombosis. Unless they are at high risk for significant bleeding, patients should have thromboembolic deterrent hose and sequential compression devices as well as prophylactic doses of heparin or low-molecular-weight heparin. Patients at very high risk may be treated with warfarin postoperatively.
- Aggressive physical therapy is necessary for postoperative recovery. All patients should have a physical therapy consultation and ordered to be out of bed three times a day unless otherwise specified by the orthopedic consultant. The orthopedic consultant will indicate the weight-bearing status of the affected extremity. It is useful to think of the elderly orthopedic patient as a shark; they must keep moving.
- Orthopedic procedures can result in significant pain. Adequate pain control is important to allow postoperative mobilization and physical therapy.

Otolaryngology

Neel Bhatt, Collin Chen, Jennifer Gross,
Heidi E. L'Esperance, Judith Lieu, and Peter M. Vila

AIRWAY EMERGENCIES

- **In the event of an airway emergency, don't panic!** But do remember, A is the first and most important part of your ABC's (airway, breathing, and circulation) assessment of the patient. **Always call a consult or the airway pager if you need assistance!** You can totally panic later.

- Quickly assess the patient. Look for signs of respiratory distress and airway compromise (e.g., noisy breathing, increased work of breathing, decreased responsiveness, inability to exchange air). If the patient is crumping and needs support, assess what would be most useful:

  - Oxygen support in order of invasiveness: nasal cannula < face mask < non-rebreather < bilevel positive airway pressure < intubation

  - Intubation is a learned skill. Each attempt can cause airway swelling, and it is vital that an airway be established quickly once this road is attempted. **Don't hesitate to call the difficult airway pager if you run into trouble.** You can't be credibly criticized for being cautious in this circumstance.

  - If there is difficulty with intubation, and the patient cannot be bag-mask ventilated (likely due to obstruction), **YOU should take slow, steady breaths and calm down.** Then think of surgical airway (cricothyroidotomy or slash tracheostomy) at the same time you are calling the difficult airway pager.

- If you have a patient with a hole in his/her neck, ask family/providers if the patient has a tracheotomy versus T-tube versus total laryngectomy. Just what every intern wants to see, a hole in the patient's neck.

  - Tracheotomy tube: It is often possible to intubate these patients orally or nasally if the trach is difficult to replace.

  - T-tube: Remove T-tube and insert breathing tube via neck.

  - Total laryngectomy: The oropharynx and trachea are no longer in communication; the patient is solely a **neck breather.** You can often slide an endotracheal tube through the hole in the neck (aka stoma). If the stoma is too small, find the tract and use a set of curved Kelly clamps to dilate the tract and insert the tube. Now doesn't that sound like fun!

- The fun just keeps coming... If you have a tracheostomy patient with a large amount of bleeding around the trach site, place a cuffed trach into the stoma and inflate the cuff. This maneuver will prevent blood from going down into the lungs and save the patient's life.

- **History**
  - Respiratory distress: onset, duration, progression, and severity. Has this happened before? Known history of angioedema?
  - Voice or swallowing changes?
  - Recent weight loss or new neck masses? History of smoking?
  - History of prior intubation or trauma to the head and neck?
  - Surgical history or radiation treatment? Tracheostomy?
  - New medications, particularly angiotensin converting enzyme (ACE) inhibitor use.
  - Allergies? Could this be an episode of anaphylaxis?

- **Physical examination**
  - Is there stertor (snoring sound with breathing)? Yeah, I've never heard of that word either. This is a sign of upper airway obstruction above the larynx.
  - Is there stridor (high-pitched, noisy breathing usually on inspiration)? This I've heard of. This sign of upper airway obstruction is due to turbulent airflow at or above the level of the vocal cords.
    - **Beware, the degree of stridor may not necessarily indicate the severity of obstruction!**
    - Inspiratory and expiratory (biphasic) stridor usually indicates obstruction just below or at the level of the vocal cords.
  - Is there wheezing (high-pitched, softer quality, usually on exhalation)? This is a sign of lower airway obstruction.
  - **Pulse oximetry is not a good marker for gauging severity of respiratory distress.** In a healthy individual, you often need several minutes of apnea before this oxygen saturation will start to fall.
  - Assess for increased work of breathing including use of accessory muscles, suprasternal/subcostal retractions, tachypnea, or decreased responsiveness from exhaustion.

- Facial or oral cavity swelling? Be sure to check the tongue and the floor of mouth.
- Is there a muffled or "hot potato" voice? This suggests oropharynx (base of tongue/tonsils) involvement.
- Is there coughing or choking? This sign suggests vocal cord involvement.
- Be sure to evaluate the tracheostomy or laryngectomy stoma if the patient has one. Check to see if the trach tube is properly in place and there is no obstructive lesion, mucous plug, or tracheal bleeding.

- **Evaluation**
  - Potentially helpful lab tests include arterial blood gases and complete blood count (if bleeding is present).
  - If there is concern for airway obstruction you cannot see, consider ordering one of the following if testing can be performed without compromising patient safety:
    - Portable neck film or chest radiograph
    - CT neck. **Don't send a patient in acute respiratory distress to the CT scanner.** You definitely won't make any friends doing this and, chances are, you'll get yelled at. **Secure an airway FIRST!**
    - Direct visualization by your friendly otolaryngology team, in the form of fiberoptic laryngoscopy.

- **Diagnosis**
  - Foreign body: This should be clear by history. Imaging may/may not show anything (e.g., a toy plane would show up on a radiograph but a carrot or hunk of chicken may not).
  - Trauma: Could have a hyoid/thyroid cartilage fracture or cervical spine fracture. Ouch!
  - Hematoma from trauma or prior surgery (e.g., thyroidectomy).
  - Airway burns: Recent exposure to house fire, etc. The patient will often have soot in nares, mouth, and/or airway. Edema is at worst from hours to days after initial injury, so if you are concerned, observe.
  - Angioedema: Often secondary to an allergy or increased bradykinin (ACE inhibitor or C1 esterase inhibitor deficiency). Swelling is often unilateral and evolves over time.
  - Anaphylaxis: Type I hypersensitivity reaction mediated by IgE and eosinophils. Swelling is often bilateral and accompanied by hypotension, rash, or wheezing.

- Infection/abscess: Don't forget Ludwig angina, which can present with rapid floor of mouth swelling, usually from a tooth abscess. Really, who could forget Ludwig? Angina, from the Latin for strangling of chocking.
- Vocal cord paralysis: Patients will likely also have breathy hoarseness and/or dysphagia; may have had a recent neck or chest surgery, intubation, or recent upper respiratory tract infection.
- Neoplasm: Can be associated with a history of tobacco use, dysphagia, and/or a new neck mass.

- **Treatment**
  - Foreign body: May need to be retrieved by otolaryngology, gastroenterology, or pulmonary.
  - Airway trauma: Treatment based on extent of trauma; may need operative repair.
  - Hematoma: May need to be evacuated. If in a post-op patient, be sure to contact the surgeon who performed the initial surgery.
  - Angioedema: Consider use of dexamethasone versus methyl-prednisolone ± H2-blocker (e.g., famotidine) ± nonselective antihistamine (e.g., diphenhydramine) ± fresh frozen plasma. Stop ACE inhibitor or angiotensin receptor blocker if on these medications.
  - Hereditary angioedema: Consider use of 2 units of fresh frozen plasma to replace depleted factors, C1 inhibitor concentrate, recombinant C1 inhibitor, bradykinin B2-receptor antagonist (icatibant), or kallikrein inhibitor (ecallantide) if severe episode of angioedema.
  - Anaphylaxis: Administer epinephrine, diphenhydramine, famotidine, and dexamethasone or methylprednisolone. Give intravenous (IV) fluids to support blood pressure.
  - If the patient is obtunded (Glasgow coma scale <8), intubate.
  - Oxygen support may be beneficial regardless of measured oxygen saturations, which may drop precipitously when complete airway obstruction or respiratory exhaustion occurs. **Do not let pulse oximeter readings override clinical examination of a stridulous patient.**
    - **Total laryngectomy patients are neck breathers only!** If you are giving them oxygen, it must be **through the neck stoma** and not the mouth!
    - If a tracheostomy patient in distress is not improving with oxygen through the trach tube, he/she may need oxygen through the mouth if there is obstruction in the trach

tube. When in doubt, you can always place oxygen on both the mouth and the trach.

- Humidified air helps to thin secretions and prevent crust formation. Use a face mask or face tent rather than nasal cannula if possible, especially in mouth-breathers.

- Systemic corticosteroids may be used if edema is suspected. Dexamethasone 10 mg and methylprednisolone 125 mg IV are most commonly used as acute treatment.

- Nebulized racemic epinephrine works quickly, acting as a topical vasoconstrictor; however, it is short acting, and there may be a rebound effect once it dissipates. In addition, it can cause acute elevations in blood pressure, which can be problematic in some patients. If there is a lack of improvement with epinephrine, one must be concerned about a fixed structural obstruction.

- Heliox refers to an 80%:20% helium-oxygen mixture. It relies on decreased density of helium to transport oxygen past the obstructed site. Usually used as a temporizing measure.

- Nasopharyngeal airway (nasal trumpet) is beneficial for patients with oropharyngeal obstruction but normal respiratory drive. It provides support to the airway at the soft palate and base of the tongue.

- Likewise, an oropharyngeal airway may treat ventilatory obstruction due to a relaxed tongue. It is not well tolerated in fully conscious patients.

- Transoral intubation is the standard for airway management. Contraindications include C-spine fractures and some types of laryngeal or tracheal trauma. The laryngeal mask airway (LMA) is another option for emergent airway management, especially as a temporizing measure. Use of this device is becoming more widespread and has the advantage of being placed without direct laryngoscopy. Endotracheal tubes can also be passed through some types of LMAs. **Consult otolaryngology when a difficult intubation is anticipated** (and/or a fiberoptic intubation would be preferred) or if a surgical airway is needed!

TRACHEOSTOMY

- **Indications**
  - There are numerous indications for tracheostomy. They include obstructed upper airway (e.g., bilateral vocal fold paralysis, laryngeal cancer), extended transoral intubation, and need for pulmonary toilet in patients who aspirate or are unable to handle their secretions. Mmm… sputum.

- In the case of extended transoral intubation, the optimal timing for a tracheostomy is controversial; however, earlier intervention has beneficial effects for critically ill patients. If long-term intubation is probable, then a tracheostomy is justified. In some patients with neuromuscular disorders or severe neurologic injury in which long-term ventilatory support is anticipated, earlier tracheostomy may be indicated.

- **History**
  - Usually, another team (e.g., ICU) requests a tracheostomy. What is their precise reason for wanting a tracheostomy?
  - You should know why the team has decided this patient needs a trach and confirm this with the patient and **his/her family.** Oftentimes the patient will be nonverbal, so you will have to talk to a family member or healthcare proxy.

- **Physical examination**
  - Pay careful attention to the neck anatomy—large, deep necks will make the procedure considerably more difficult (and is more dangerous postoperatively if the trach tube becomes dislodged).
  - Look and palpate for airway landmarks, including the cricoid cartilage, thyroid cartilage, and trachea.
  - Central venous catheters may need to be moved to other sites prior to the procedure. Excessive tracheal secretions on a central line in the internal jugular vein can cause infections, and tracheotomy ties may compress and clot off the catheter, but they are not hard contraindications.
  - Is the patient intubated already?

- **Evaluation**
  - Patients with bleeding issues or on anticoagulation (including ASA) are at higher risk of both intraoperative and postoperative hemorrhage. Reverse or discontinue anticoagulation, if possible. If it can't be stopped, discuss this with your attending as to whether the procedure will occur.
  - Patients with high peak airway pressures are at greater risk for ventilatory complications because of leakage of air around the tracheostomy tube and the need for excessive cuff pressures to maintain a seal.
  - Prognosis is a key component of discussion with the family regarding the purposes of a tracheostomy. Assistance with long ventilator weans is an appropriate indication, as is palliation of airway obstruction in end-of-life situations.

- **Treatment**
  - Two types of tracheostomy may be performed: **open surgical tracheostomy** (performed in the operating room) or **bedside percutaneous dilational tracheostomy** (PDT). PDT avoids transporting a critically ill patient out of the ICU but may be prone to complications in some patients (e.g., obese or prior neck surgery). The choice of procedure is dependent on patient characteristics, as well as the experience and preference of the surgeon.
  - Types of tracheostomy tubes: Tubes come in metal or plastic varieties. Shiley, Bivona, and Portex brand tubes are plastic and come with or without cuffs. Cuffs are necessary when ventilatory support is needed and are always used as the initial tracheostomy tube. Jackson tubes are metal and are not cuffed. After the tracheostomy, the tube is kept undisturbed for 3 to 7 days to allow for formation of a well-healed tract. At this point, the original tube is changed to either a similar cuffed tube or a cuffless tube if ventilatory support is not required.
  - **For all patients with a tracheostomy**
    - Always have appropriate spare tracheostomy tubes immediately available in the patient's room and have the obturator secured to the foot of the bed where it is easily accessible. The obturator is the metal or plastic inner piece that facilitates reinsertion of the tracheostomy tube. Nurses and physicians caring for these patients should know its location and have immediate access to it.
    - Patient should wear a high-humidity trach collar to thin secretions.
    - Always have suction catheters available at the bedside for immediate use.
    - Always have an immediately visible sign (e.g., red, yellow, or green airway signs) at the bedside describing the airway anatomy (e.g., total laryngectomy, partially obstructed, not obstructed) detailing what is safe to do in an emergency to obtain a stable airway.
    - See the pattern here? **The aforementioned things are not negotiable and will save lives**.
  - Posttracheostomy care: The first tracheostomy tube change occurs 3 to 7 days postoperatively to ensure a well-healed tract has formed and is safe. In most cases, further tracheostomy changes can be performed by nursing staff on the floors or

by the patient/family upon discharge. Frequent cleaning or changing of the inner cannula is recommended to prevent obstruction by crusting (typically at least three times per day).

- **Dislodged tracheostomy tube**: If the tracheostomy tube comes out, first assess the stability of the patient and **don't panic!**

  - If the patient is stable and comfortable, you may attempt to reinsert the tracheostomy tube. Using a small Kelly clamp to retract the skin, along with a bright light source, may give a better view of the tract. You may reinsert the tube with the aid of the obturator and resecure the collar to prevent further dislodgement. Occasionally, passing the tracheostomy tube over a Foley catheter, nasogastric tube, or suction catheter will do the trick.

  - **If the patient is in respiratory distress, call (or have someone else call) the ENT on-call or the difficult airway team immediately.** If the tracheostomy tube is in place but there is no airflow, it is likely in a false tract. Removing the tube and reattempting with the methods mentioned will usually allow for correct placement. If in proper position, you should be able to feel the expired airflow through the tracheostomy tube. A tracheal suction catheter should pass easily into the trachea via the tube. Finally, a flexible fiber-optic scope can be advanced through the tracheostomy tube to confirm placement into the airway (you should see tracheal rings if the tube is in place).

  - **If tracheostomy tube insertion is not possible or unsuccessful and the patient is decompensating, transoral endotracheal intubation may be an option.** Patients with tracheostomy tubes have variable degrees of upper airway patency. In the case of a patent or even a partially obstructed upper airway, transoral endotracheal intubation can be performed. **With a completely obstructed upper airway, however, transoral intubation should not be attempted. This group includes patients with a total laryngectomy.**

EPISTAXIS

- Undoubtedly during the course of your training, whatever your specialty, you will be called by a frantic nurse or other provider for someone with a bloody nose. As always, avoid freaking out; this generally never helps, with anything. Another thing that doesn't help, having the patient lay down on their back with an ice cube in their belly button.

- Although a slow dribble may present an annoyance to the patient, and something a little more brisk may present a challenge to control for even the most experienced provider, **this is rarely life-threatening** if caught early but is extremely disconcerting for the patient and can lead to severe aspiration and death if left unchecked long enough.

- Grab a bottle of oxymetazoline (i.e., Afrin), spray the patient's nose with a couple of big squirts, pinch the floppy part at the patient's nostrils (a.k.a. the nasal ala) firmly, sit the patient upright so that the blood isn't going down their throat, and then begin asking questions. Now how easy is that?

- **History**

  - **The first question to ask the physician consulting you on the phone is this: what has been tried in order to control the bleeding?** If the answer is nothing, then have them squirt lots of Afrin in both sides of the nose, sit the patient up, and have them hold pressure. This will buy you time while you get to the bedside.

  - Once at the bedside, you can decide how much of a history to get immediately depending on whether the patient is young versus old, drenched in blood (oh joy!) versus having a small bleed, etc. The answers to these questions will dictate how extensive a history you will be taking, because if their nose is gushing blood, you will be less inclined to ask questions and more inclined to take action. We call this situational awareness. Don't worry, you got this!

  - Other important information to gather

    - How long has the nose been bleeding? How much blood? Most patients will say "a lot" no matter what, but try to get them to quantify it using terms they understand, such as a bloody tissue versus a solo cup versus a coffee mug.

    - What things have been tried? (Afrin, pressure, etc.)

    - How did the current episode start?

    - History of nasal trauma. Ask about digital trauma (i.e., nose picking) or trauma from nasal cannula or feeding tube use, history of cocaine use. Your mother always told you not to pick your nose!

    - History of coagulopathy, a vascular disorder, renal disease, hepatic dysfunction, or HIV

- Is the patient on aspirin or other antiplatelet agents, warfarin, or other anticoagulants?
- **Physical examination**
  - Vital signs: Pay attention to blood pressure, as this may need to be brought down before you try anything invasive.
  - Side of the nose that is bleeding and amount of bleeding
  - Blood in the back of the throat (the oropharynx) and/or coming from the mouth
  - Able to maintain airway versus need for more urgent intervention
  - General physical exam and head and neck exam
- **Differential diagnosis**
  - Digital trauma (polite term of plain old nose picking)
  - Trauma from nasal cannula, Dobhoff tube placement, or other nasally placed item
  - Adverse effect of anticoagulation and/or antiplatelet therapy
  - Severe hypertension
  - Foreign body (the much-discussed green crayon)
  - Hereditary hemorrhagic telangiectasia (HHT): Usually patients will know this or report a history of recurrent nosebleeds or family members with the same. You will see telangiectasias on the lips and tongue in addition to the nose.
  - HIV/AIDs: Sometimes initial presentation is a profuse nosebleed that won't stop as HIV can cause thrombocytopenia.
  - Cocaine use: May also have history of other substance abuse. Snortin' some coke lines.
  - Cirrhosis due to side effect of thrombocytopenia and low coagulation factors
  - Renal failure: Elevated blood urea nitrogen can inhibit platelet function.
  - Hemophilia, um, duh.
  - von Willebrand disease and nosebleeds are classic.
  - Granulomatosis with polyangiitis (a.k.a. Wegener granulomatosis).
  - Septal perforation: as this crusts can cause recurrent bouts of epistaxis.
  - Aging/thinning of mucosa: Nose will otherwise appear to have dry and shiny mucosa.
  - Malignancy: nasopharyngeal carcinoma, juvenile angiofibroma (think about this in an adolescent male), lymphoma, and other sinonasal malignancies

- **Treatment**
  - After using oxymetazoline and holding pressure for 15 minutes, you note that the patient is still bleeding. What next? Panic? Absolutely not! You're as cool as a cucumber.
    - Control underlying factors for bleeding, i.e., get the patient's blood pressure controlled, and work toward normalizing their platelets and/or clotting factors.
    - Try a different method to stop bleeding.
      - If you can see a discrete source of bleeding, you can cauterize this with silver nitrate (messy and painful).
      - If the patient has HHT or abnormal coagulation and/ or platelets, consider attempting a nonpressure form of epistaxis control such as Hemaderm, Floseal, or other topical clotting agent since these patients have a tendency to bleed when packing materials are removed. These agents work best after suctioning out blood and clots and applying them directly to the mucosa.
      - Pack the nose with a 7.5 cm Rapid Rhino, Merocel sponge, Surgicel wrapped Gelfoam, or whatever the nasal packing du jour is at your institution.
      - If you decide to go this route, consider putting the patient on anti-Staph antibiotics to prevent toxic shock.
      - When placing, glide the object along the floor of the nose. Never force these objects in!
      - If bilateral packing is required, consider ICU admission due to risk of vagal stimulation resulting in hypotension.
    - **Don't use plain gauze, paper towels, or facial tissue in the nose**—these can cause further nasal damage and debride the septum. Many a well-meaning intern or nurse has worsened the bleeding by doing so!
    - If you have tried various methods and they have all failed, it may be time to consider something more invasive… Call for help!
  - Intubation for airway protection with packing of nasal and/ or oral cavities
  - Sphenopalatine artery (SPA) ligation by your friendly otolaryngology service
  - Internal maxillary artery embolization by interventional radiology
  - Phew. The bleeding is controlled. Great job. But what next?

- Schedule follow-up to have the nasal packing removed in 3 to 5 days and get a proper scope exam by an otolaryngologist for the patient if the cause of bleeding unclear.
- Control factors that could cause rebleeding and avoiding further nasal trauma
- Instruct patient to not blow the nose (easier said than done), sneeze with the mouth open, and avoid straining with bowel movements.
- Begin patient on nasal moisture regimen such as ocean nasal spray, high-humidity face tent, and some Vaseline or Ayr (saline) gel if going home.
- Consider using Afrin twice daily for 3 days only—**do not use Afrin for more than 3 days!**
- If mass or malignancy is high on differential, consider imaging to further evaluate the lesion and consult otolaryngology to obtain a biopsy.

ACUTE SINUSITIS

- Before we get into the heavy stuff, it's important to understand that just like interns, the poor sinuses often get mistakenly blamed for a lot of random things. You may hear, "doc my sinuses are acting up!" ...or "I've got a case of the sinuses!" Many times, patients will interchangeably use the word "sinus" when they really mean "nose" (the rhinus). For example, in the case of nasal congestion or a runny nose, you may hear, "my sinuses are clogged up again!" Upon asking the patient to describe their symptoms further, a more accurate description may be clear rhinorrhea associated with difficulty breathing through the nose, with no facial tenderness, pressure, or purulent drainage. Make sure you get an accurate history and description of the symptoms so that you get a good idea of what's actually bothering the patient.

- Many times, you will find incidental radiologic evidence of "sinusitis" after a head CT or MRI. More often than not, the patient has no sinus complaints and there are no abnormalities on exam to warrant treatment. This is where a more detailed history including allergies, nasal medications, previous sinus surgeries, and severity will shed light on the diagnosis. If you suspect the patient has uncomplicated bacterial sinusitis, you can offer either watchful waiting or treat with antibiotics (remember, the antibiotic of choice is amoxicillin with or without clavulanate for 5-10 d). Uncomplicated sinusitis is not an ENT emergency. Feel free to have these patients follow up in ENT clinic.

- Time for the heavy stuff. Most of the time, the sinuses play nice and don't cause major problems beyond frequent urgent care visits. However, there are certain situations where the sinuses are the cause of medical emergencies and warrant immediate ENT evaluation.

Complicated Acute Sinusitis

- Complicated acute sinusitis is an emergency when the infection has extended past the sinuses to involve intraorbital or intracranial structures. **If this is suspected or confirmed, call a consultant immediately!**
- **History**
    - Duration of sinusitis symptoms: Usually these patients have the acute sinusitis history but never improved and the symptoms only became worse. They may have eye pain, vision changes, mental status changes, cranial nerve deficits (eye and skull base involvement is always abnormal).
    - Ask what antibiotics they have been treated with in the past or if they have had surgery.
    - Predisposing factors include malnutrition, diabetes, chemotherapy, long-term corticosteroids, allergic rhinitis, immunodeficiency states, environmental exposures, and the presence of nasogastric tube.
- **Physical examination**
    - Perform a full head and neck exam.
    - Assess for meningeal signs.
    - Look for orbital signs (e.g., proptosis, chemosis, ophthalmoplegia, vision loss).
    - Test for other cranial nerve involvement such as sensation changes in the face.
- **Evaluation:** High-resolution maxillofacial CT (with coronal cuts) with contrast to assess for subperiosteal/orbital abscess. Head CT with contrast may also be indicated to look for intracranial involvement.
- **Treatment**
    - An ophthalmology consult is required if there is suspected orbital involvement. They will be able to document pressures and visual acuity changes that determine the need for intervention.
    - IV antibiotics (including anaerobic coverage)
    - Copious use of saline (Ocean) nasal spray (e.g., q1h while awake) and 3 days of oxymetazoline to aid in decongesting the nose

- IV steroids (dexamethasone 10 mg or methylprednisolone 125 mg) to help diminish edema around orbits and reduce optic nerve damage
- Surgery (functional endoscopic sinus surgery or external surgical drainage) is definitive therapy to drain abscess and sinuses.
- If optic nerve damage is imminent because of intraorbital abscess, then immediate lateral canthotomy with tendon cantholysis should be done to decrease intraocular pressure. And doesn't that sound like fun!

Invasive Fungal Sinusitis

- First, it is important to distinguish invasive fulminant fungal sinusitis from allergic fungal sinusitis.
  - **Allergic fungal sinusitis** is a common allergic reaction to fungi in the environment. It occurs in immunocompetent hosts, often with history of allergic rhinitis, and manifests as thick fungal debris and mucin in the sinus cavities.
  - In contrast, **invasive fungal sinusitis** occurs in immunocompromised patients and manifests as rapidly progressive fungal infection starting in the nasal cavity or sinuses and invading bony and surrounding soft tissue structures.
- **History**
  - Occurs in immunocompromised patients such as diabetic ketoacidosis, neutropenia (chemotherapy, bone marrow or solid organ transplant, leukemia), and advanced AIDS. Find out if your patient has any of these.
  - These patients are usually hospitalized and very sick and cannot provide a detailed history; thus, early clinical suspicion is key to diagnosis and treatment.
- **Physical examination**
  - Common things in this condition: fevers, purulent nasal drainage, headache, and mental status changes
  - During your exam, look into the nose with an otoscope or nasal speculum and you may see black ulcers or spots on the septum or turbinates. **If you see this, call an ENT immediately!**
- **Evaluation**
  - Find and characterize the source of the immunosuppression (e.g., blood glucose, neutrophil count, HIV test).
  - Imaging with maxillofacial CT without contrast will show bony destruction.

- MRI with contrast will assess for invasion into masticator space, periorbital fat, pterygopalatine fossa.
- ENT will perform an endoscopic exam and biopsy suspicious necrotic tissue to confirm invasive fungal infection.
- **Treatment**
  - The most effective treatment for these patients is reversal of their immunocompromised states. Until that occurs, they will benefit from debridement of their nasal cavity and sinuses in the operating room by ENT, sometimes multiple trips to the operating room.
  - Systemic IV antifungals should also be administered.

VERTIGO

- Fortunately, emergencies involving vertigo are rare and include the following (hopefully realize that none of them are actually ENT issues):
  - **Neurovascular issues** (e.g., Wallenberg lateral medullary syndrome, lateral pontomedullary syndrome, cerebellar hemorrhage, cerebellar infarction, vertebrobasilar insufficiency)
  - **Sudden sensorineural hearing loss** is an emergency and is occasionally associated with vertigo.
- **History**
  - Your job is to decide whether the dizziness is due to a central (call Neuro) or a peripheral cause (call ENT).
  - Sensation and duration of dizziness (important to clarify room-spinning vertigo vs. disequilibrium associated with migraine vs. chronic imbalance)
  - Immediate versus progressive onset versus situational onset (triggers such as changes in head position suggestive of benign positional vertigo versus standing from sitting position suggestive of orthostatic hypotension or cardiac cause)
  - Otologic symptoms (e.g., hearing loss, otalgia, otorrhea, tinnitus)
  - Associated neurologic symptoms including headache, visual changes, unilateral weakness, dysarthria, dysphagia, paresthesias, nausea/vomiting
  - History of vascular problems including diabetes mellitus complications, stroke, or myocardial infarction
  - New or recently started medications

- Recent head trauma
- Changes in diet cause increased symptoms (e.g., increased salt load or caffeine, cheeses, wine).
- Family history of dizziness (e.g., otosclerosis, CHARGE syndrome). Otosclerosis tends to run in families. CHARGE stands for Coloboma, Heart defects, Atresia choanae, Retardation of growth and/or development, Genital and/or urinary abnormalities, Ear abnormalities and deafness. This rare syndrome is often associated with mutations in the CHD7 gene and was mentioned just to impress you. What's a coloboma anyway? A fancy word for a hole in the eye.
- Psychiatric history
- **Physical examination**
  - Head: Look for evidence of trauma from a recent fall, facial asymmetry.
  - Ears: Perform a thorough otologic exam. Check external ear for skin changes (e.g., erythema, swelling, vesicles), external auditory canal (look for cerumen impaction or foreign bodies, including gross things such as cockroaches, or evidence of trauma), appearance and patency of tympanic membrane (intact vs. perforated), middle ear (aerated vs. fluid filled), pneumatic otoscopy (blow air into ear canal while sealed to check for tympanic membrane movement).
  - Neurological exam (the hard part):
    - Nystagmus is defined by horizontal versus vertical (the direction of the fast phase), spontaneous versus gaze-evoked, fatigable versus nonfatigable, and visual fixation suppression of the vestibule-ocular reflex (which suggests a peripheral lesion). Perform the Dix-Hallpike maneuver to look for torsional upbeating nystagmus, which is most commonly seen with posterior canal benign positional vertigo.
    - Head thrust/impulse test: Check for a catchup saccade, suggestive of unilateral vestibular hypofunction.
    - Hearing loss: Perform the Weber and Rinne tests with 512 Hz tuning fork (the smaller one without the thingies on the end). Rinne (pronounced RIN-na, like pinna) was a German otolaryngologist, hence the pronunciation. Pronouncing it like "Renée" (as in Renée Zellweger) is a quick and easy way to get a laugh out of your ENT colleagues. It is important not to sound stupid.

- Also look for other potentially important neurologic findings such as diplopia, dysarthria, drop attacks, decreased visual acuity, dysphagia, loss of pain/temperature sensation, loss of motor control, Horner syndrome (i.e., ptosis, miosis, anhidrosis), and nuchal rigidity. We presume you know how to pronounce Horner.

- **Evaluation**
  - Usually, history and physical examination will give you the diagnosis if it is truly an ENT-related problem.
  - Rule out medical causes including hypotension or hypertension, cardiac arrhythmias, endocrine abnormalities.
  - May need CT/MRI or cerebral angiogram depending on suspected etiology.
  - Neurology consultation if evidence of central cause of vertigo or other associated symptoms suggestive of stroke
  - Audiogram if concern for acute hearing loss

- **Diagnosis**
  - Most common etiologies are benign paroxysmal positional vertigo (BPPV), Ménière disease (pretty sure that guy was French), migraine-associated vertigo, and vestibular neuritis.
  - BPPV is typically associated with changes in head position (turning head while lying in bed), **vertigo lasts seconds to minutes**, no associated hearing loss or other symptoms.
  - Ménière disease has **vertigo that lasts hours**, often associated with intermittent hearing loss, may have drop attacks in severe cases, and can be associated with changes in diet (i.e., increased salt load).
  - Migraine-associated vertigo (a.k.a., vertiginous migraine or vestibular migraine) **lasts minutes to hours**, is associated with migraine ± aura, and can also be associated with certain food/drink triggers (e.g., wine, caffeine, cheese, chocolate).
  - Vestibular neuritis causes **vertigo that lasts days**, is often preceded by a viral prodrome, and can be associated with tinnitus.

- **Treatment**
  - For most ENT-related causes of vertigo (e.g., BPPV, Ménière disease, vestibular neuritis, migraine-associated vertigo), treatment in the acute setting consists of supportive care.
  - Epley maneuver for otolith repositioning: If you believe the patient has BPPV, you can cure the patient with an Epley! The Dix-Hallpike maneuver is the first step of the Epley maneuver

for the affected ear. It usually takes more than one treatment to completely resolve the problem. Counsel the patient that they may have some disequilibrium afterward that can last several days, and they should sleep upright the first night if possible.

- Short-term symptomatic treatment may include vestibular suppressants such as:
  - Meclizine 12.5 to 25 mg PO q8h PRN
  - Prochlorperazine suppositories 25 mg q6h PRN
  - Diazepam 2 to 10 mg PO q6h PRN
  - For severe cases, diazepam 5 to 10 mg IM or droperidol 2.5 mg IM
  - **Remember that these are only short-term treatments** to help patient with the acute (and usually most severe) part of the vertigo. The longer they stay on these medications, the longer it takes for their brain to adjust, and the whole process is prolonged. Thus, think very hard about whether the patient needs such medications. These are just not long-term treatments.
  - Can also include antiemetics such as ondansetron IV or metoclopramide IV.
- Consider oral versus intratympanic steroids for acute sensorineural hearing loss (avoid oral if patient is diabetic or has a history of problems with oral steroids such as mood changes).

Psychiatry

27

Gemma Espejo and Brendan O'Connor

GENERAL GUIDELINES

- Prior to calling a consult, ask if the patient is willing to speak with psychiatry service. The patient has the right to refuse psychiatric consultation unless:
    - There is concern about the patient being a danger to himself/herself or others
    - There is concern about the patient's ability to make medical decisions
- Obtain basic information and key psychiatric history prior to calling the consult: age, gender, previous psychiatric diagnoses, current treatment (including if a patient has a current outpatient psychiatrist), recent substance use, current suicide ideation and plan, current psychosis, current agitation, and sensorium (alert and oriented to self, location, date).
- Having a clear question for the consult service will best serve your patient care needs. Asking for a generic "psych eval" is not usually very productive. Following are appropriate examples of well-defined consultations:
    - A 50-year-old man with a history of depression here for chronic obstructive pulmonary disease exacerbation, currently endorsing suicide ideation with plan to hang himself. We are wondering if psychiatric admission is appropriate because of safety concerns.
    - A 35-year-old woman with a history of schizophrenia here for abdominal pain, currently on risperidone 4 mg, who appears actively psychotic. We are consulting for medication recommendations and possible evaluation for admission.
    - A 45-year-old man with a history of phencyclidine (PCP) use, urine drug screen (UDS) pending, here for sepsis in setting of multiple ulcers. He is currently agitated and threatening staff. We want recommendations for pharmacologic treatment of agitation.

SUICIDALITY

Assessment

- Suicidal ideation is a symptom and not indicative of a specific psychiatric diagnosis—it may be present in patients with depression, schizophrenia, bipolar disorder, substance use disorders, etc.
- Ask **explicitly** about suicide ideation. Bringing up suicide ideation will not cause or "plant" the idea.
- If the patient endorses suicide ideation, ask about specific plan and his/her level of intent.
- There may be concern for suicide ideation even if the patient denies such ideation. Be vigilant if:
  - Collateral sources express concern for suicide ideation
  - The patient appears guarded or makes noncommittal statements when directly asked about suicidal thoughts

Management

- If there are concerns that the patient may act on suicidal thoughts, it may be appropriate to order one-to-one observation pending full psychiatric consultation.
- If a patient is suicidal and a psychiatric consult has been called, do not discharge the patient from medical unit prior to clearance from the psychiatric team. Transfer to psychiatry may be appropriate on a voluntary or even involuntary basis.

AGITATION

- Agitation may occur in several neuropsychiatric disorders. In inpatient settings, these are most commonly delirium, substance use disorders, personality disorders, and psychotic disorders.
- It may be appropriate to call security for acute situations before the arrival of psychiatric consult service.
- Oral and parenteral antipsychotics are first-line treatment for severe agitation not amenable to redirection or less invasive forms of restriction. Please see Table 27-1 for commonly used medications for acute agitation.
- Physical or chemical interventions may be appropriate if verbal redirection fails. Choosing a combination of approaches (see Figure 27-1) should be based on individualized risks and benefits. Frequent reassessment for appropriate level of restraints necessary for safety and documentation of interventions is important.

TABLE 27-1 COMMONLY USED MEDICATIONS FOR ACUTE AGITATION

Medication	Dosage	Formulations	Considerations
Haloperidol (Haldol)	5 mg every 4-6 h Avoid >20 mg IM in a 24-h period	PO, IM, IV	• Use lactate form. Haldol comes in decanoate form—long-acting injections for maintenance treatment (typically given once a month). • Avoid IV because of risk of Torsades de Pointes. • Do not use in patients with Parkinson disease. • Higher risk of extrapyramidal symptoms (EPS) than atypical antipsychotics such as olanzapine or ziprasidone • Can be coadministered with benzodiazepines
Chlorpromazine (Thorazine)	25-50 mg IM every 4-6 h	PO, IM	• Highly anticholinergic • Look out for postural hypotension. • Lower doses/avoid in the elderly. • Lower risk of EPS
Olanzapine (Zyprexa)	5-10 mg IM every 6 h Avoid >30 mg in a 24-h period	PO (including disintegrating tablet), IM	• Avoid coadministration with benzodiazepines when given IM.
Ziprasidone (Geodon)	10-20 mg IM every 2-4 h Maximal dose 40 mg IM in 24-h period	PO, IM	• Caution in renal failure • Associated with QTc prolongation
Lorazepam (Ativan)	1-2 mg every 4 h	PO, IM, IV	• Can be used with haloperidol • Avoid in delirium.

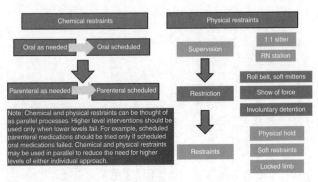

Figure 27-1. Chemical and physical restraints.

- Clinical pearls
  - If you have concerns about your own safety, ask another staff member or security to be present for interview.
  - If the situation escalates, leave the room. It is usually not possible to reason with an agitated patient, and repeated attempts to do so often worsen the situation.

DELIRIUM

Assessment

- Delirium consists of impaired attention and awareness associated with other cognitive disturbances (i.e., problems with orientation, language, memory, perception, etc.).
- Can present with numerous psychiatric symptoms mimicking different disorders.
- Acute onset (hours to days)
- Fluctuation: waxing/waning accompanied by change in cognition that cannot be better explained by another neurocognitive disorder, such as dementia. Patients may be able to correctly report name and date during morning rounds but get date wrong when evaluated later in the day.
- Can be hypoactive or hyperactive; hypoactive forms are usually more common.
- Can indicate a medical emergency.
- Initial examination and workup:

- At minimum, check if a patient can accurately state name, location, time of day, and date. It is appropriate to check for orientation with each encounter, as fluctuation is a key feature of delirium.
- Know the patient's baseline. Examples of questions to ask collateral informants:
  - Can the patient usually tell you the month/year/time of day?
  - Can the patient usually do simple math calculations in his/her head?
  - Can the patient usually follow along when other people are talking?
- Workup of organic causes usually includes basic lab tests, e.g., complete blood count, complete metabolic panel, urinalysis, and UDS. Other tests are often indicated depending on the clinical situation. These can include an arterial blood gas, serum ammonia, EEG, brain imaging, and cerebrospinal fluid studies.
- Consider substance intoxication and withdrawal.

Management

- Low-dose antipsychotics
- Avoid benzodiazepines (unless there is concern for benzodiazepine or alcohol withdrawal). Benzodiazepines can worsen symptoms of delirium.
- Limit narcotics unless medically necessary.
- Avoid anticholinergic medications.
- Consider psychiatric consultation for behavioral management.

PSYCHOSIS

- Definition: Neuropsychiatric disturbance characterized by the presence of hallucinations, delusions, disorganized thought, and/or disorganized behavior.
- Psychosis can be present in patients with major depressive disorder, bipolar disorder, schizophrenia, substance intoxication/withdrawal, and neurocognitive disorders (delirium and dementias).
  - Acute-onset psychosis in the setting of confusion can indicate delirium, which is a medical emergency. Be suspicious in the elderly and patients with severe medical illness.

- The modality of hallucinations can sometimes indicate the underlying cause:
  - Auditory hallucinations are most common in mood and psychotic disorders.
  - Visual hallucinations are more often seen in delirium, dementias, substance intoxication.
  - Olfactory/gustatory hallucinations can indicate neurologic etiologies such as seizures.
  - Tactile hallucinations are most commonly present in substance withdrawal (i.e., PCP).
- Presence of psychosis does not necessarily warrant a psychiatric consultation.
- Psychiatric consultation is indicated if there are safety concerns, if the symptoms are new, if the symptom is getting in the way of treatment, or if psychosis is impairing decision-making ability. If there are questions about medication management, a psychiatric consultation or discussion with the outpatient psychiatrist is appropriate.

CAPACITY

- Definition: ability of the patient to provide informed consent for a specific decision.
- Please see Figure 27-2 for components of capacity.

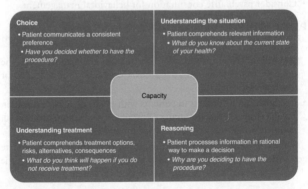

Figure 27-2. Components of capacity.

- Investigating capacity: If a patient lacks any of the four components of capacity, the patient does not have capacity to decide medical treatment.
  - For example, a patient who meets criteria for choice, understanding the situation and treatment, but is refusing thoracentesis because he/she thinks he/she will become an android if metal pierces his/her skin is not demonstrating capacity to refuse a thoracentesis because he/she does not show rational reasoning.
- If a patient does not demonstrate capacity:
  - Investigate whether the patient has a designated healthcare proxy and/or advanced directives.
    - Healthcare proxy: legal document empowering a designated person to make decisions in the event the patient cannot (i.e., a durable power of attorney)
    - Advance directives: a document providing instructions for specific situations should the patient be rendered incapacitated (i.e., living will)
  - If there is no officially designated surrogate decision-maker, state laws vary on who plays a role in making medical decisions. Contact risk management.
- There are situations in which capacity does not need to be investigated: emergency situations, court-appointed guardian, or a patient's waiver of the right to consent.
  - If a patient has a court-appointed guardian for medical decisions, **all** treatment decisions including discharge must be carried out with the consent of the guardian.
  - Only patients legally determined to be incompetent are appointed a guardian.
  - Incompetence can only be declared by a judge.
- Clinical pearls
  - Capacity **is cross-sectional**, meaning it is decision-specific and time-specific.
  - Before capacity can be assessed, patients should be given all relevant information (nature of the illness, risks, benefits, side effects, alternatives of proposed treatment) by primary teams. For example, an orthopedic surgeon can better explain the procedure and risks of an open reduction internal fixation than a psychiatrist. **Any physician can assess capacity for medical decision-making.**
  - Presence of an active psychiatric disorder does not necessarily preclude capacity, but a psychiatry consultation can be helpful in the setting of symptomatic illness.

- Other scenarios to consider psychiatric consultation are as follows:
  - Suicidal patient refusing treatment
  - Inconsistent decision-making—patient wavers
  - Disagreement between the family, patient, and/or treatment team
  - Intellectual disability

SUBSTANCE WITHDRAWAL SYNDROMES

Alcohol/Benzodiazepine Withdrawal

- Alcohol and benzodiazepine withdrawal represent clinically similar syndromes.
- Symptoms occur within a few hours to a few days and include tachycardia, diaphoresis, tremor, nausea/emesis, insomnia, psychomotor agitation, anxiety, and seizures.
- Delirium tremens is the most severe form of alcohol withdrawal with a high mortality rate. It can include altered mental status, autonomic instability (tachycardia, hypertension, hyperthermia), and perceptual disturbances (auditory, tactile, visual hallucinations).
- Treatment
  - Clinical Institute Withdrawal Assessment of Alcohol Scale, Revised (CIWA-Ar) is a standard, widely available measure for withdrawal severity once a diagnosis of alcohol or benzodiazepine withdrawal has been made.[1]
  - Many hospitals have a symptom-based order set derived from CIWA-Ar. Check with your institution and familiarize yourself with the protocol.
    - Minor withdrawal (scoring <8) is typically not treated with medication. Scores >8 are generally treated with medication administration (e.g., lorazepam 2 mg PO/IV). Scores >15 indicate severe withdrawal.[2]
    - Alternatively, chlordiazepoxide is used but is less safe in patients with liver disease.
- For benzodiazepines, medications with shorter half-lives (alprazolam) have increased risks of withdrawal than those with longer half-lives (clonazepam).

Opioid Withdrawal

- Symptoms occur within minutes to several days and may include yawning, nausea/emesis, muscle aches, lacrimation, rhinorrhea,

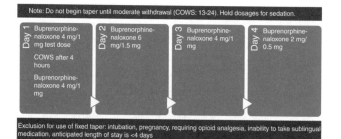

Figure 27-3. Fixed taper schedule using buprenorphine and naloxone for opioid withdrawal. COWS, Clinical Opiate Withdrawal Scale.

pupillary dilation, piloerection, diaphoresis, diarrhea, fever, insomnia, and low mood.

- Clinical Opiate Withdrawal Scale (COWS) is a standard, widely available measure for withdrawal severity—it is typically done every 4 hours.[3]
- Suboxone (buprenorphine + naloxone), methadone, or other opiates may be used for acute withdrawal.
- Please see Figure 27-3 for a sample fixed taper schedule using buprenorphine and naloxone for opioid withdrawal.
- For long-term maintenance therapy, an outpatient provider should agree to continue to prescribe controlled substances.
- Psychiatric consultation is not required for all cases of opioid withdrawal but should be considered when:
  - The patient does not respond as expected to treatment
  - There are complicated detox syndromes including comorbid withdrawal from other substances
- Other symptoms of opioid withdrawal are treatment symptomatically; please see Table 27-2.

Other Substances

The following intoxication and withdrawal syndromes are non–life-threatening, short-lived, and typically treated symptomatically.

- Stimulants (cocaine, methamphetamines)
  - Intoxication: tachycardia or bradycardia, pupillary dilations, hypertension or hypotension, diaphoresis, chills, nausea/emesis, muscular weakness, respiratory depression, chest pain,

TABLE 27-2	COMMONLY USED AS-NEEDED MEDICATIONS FOR OPIOID WITHDRAWAL	
Medication	**Dosing**	**Symptoms**
Acetaminophen	650 mg q4-6h	Pain
Clonidine	0.1 mg q8h	Autonomic dysregulation
Hyoscyamine	0.125-0.25 mg q4h	Abdominal cramps
Ibuprofen	400 mg PO q4h	Pain
Loperamide	4 mg, 2 mg after each loose stool (maximum 16 mg/d)	Diarrhea
Ondansetron	4-8 mg q6h	Nausea

cardiac arrhythmias, psychomotor agitation, dystonia, confusion, seizures, coma
  - Withdrawal: fatigue, vivid dreams, insomnia, hypersomnia, increased appetite, psychomotor slowing or agitation
- PCP
  - Intoxication: vertical or horizontal nystagmus, hypertension, tachycardia, diminished response to pain, ataxia, dysarthria, hyperacusis, muscle rigidity, seizures, coma, impulsivity, aggression
  - Withdrawal: no clear syndrome
- Cannabis
  - Intoxication: tachycardia; dry mouth; increased appetite; conjunctival injection; auditory, visual, or tactile hallucinations
  - Withdrawal: irritability, anxiety, sleep/appetite changes, abdominal pain, tremors, diaphoresis, chills, headache, fever
- Clinical pearls
  - All patients should be screened for alcohol and substance use.
  - Withdrawal from alcohol and benzodiazepines can result in death.
  - Following detox, encourage the patient to seek treatment for substance use. Social work can provide resources and referrals.

DOMESTIC VIOLENCE, RAPE, TRAUMA

- All patients should be screened for the presence of ongoing abuse.
- Physicians are mandated reporters of child abuse. Laws vary per state regarding mandated reporting of elder abuse. There are no legal requirements for spousal abuse.
- Rape victims should be evaluated by a qualified provider regarding treatment, collection of evidence, STI (sexually transmitted infection) workup.
- Most institutions have a system in place for victims of violence/abuse. Familiarize yourself with resources available at your hospital. These services typically include evaluation and referral to community support programs.
- Psychiatric consultation may be appropriate if there are acute safety concerns including suicidal ideation and homicidal ideation.

References

1. Sullivan JT, Sykora K, Schneiderman J, et al. Assessment of alcohol withdrawal: the revised Clinical Institute Withdrawal Assessment for Alcohol scale (CIWA-Ar). *Br J Addict* 1989;84:1353-7.
2. Daeppen J-B, Gache P, Landry U, et al. Symptom-triggered vs fixed-schedule doses of benzodiazepine for alcohol withdrawl. *Arch Intern Med* 2002; 162:1117-21.
3. Wesson DR, Ling W. The Clinical Opiate Withdrawal Scale (COWS). *J Psychoactive Drugs* 2003;35:253-9.

General Surgery

28

Jared M. McAllister, Jennifer Yu, and
Bradley D. Freeman

INTRODUCTION

- The following recommendations apply to most instances when calling for a surgical consultation.
- Identify yourself and the patient who needs a consultation and then clearly identify the questions you need to answer.
- Give an indication of the urgency of the consultation (i.e., stat, urgent [within a few hours], or elective [within 24 h]).
- Succinctly present the crucial information.
- State whether important radiographs have been obtained. If they are not accessible to the consultants electronically (i.e., if they were done at another hospital), provide their location.
- State whether the patient has had a recent operation, and who performed it, or whether the patient has ever been operated on for a similar or related problem, and by whom if known.
- For example: *Hi, this is Mike Smith. I am a medicine resident. I have an urgent consult regarding the management of a patient with a pulseless and cold right foot. The patient is Mr. Smith, his DOB is x/x/230 and he is located in room 230230. He is a 62-year-old diabetic man with CAD and severe PVD who...*

ACUTE ABDOMEN

- Is there badness in this belly?
- **An acute abdomen warrants immediate surgical assessment and possible emergent intervention.**
- The diagnosis of an acute abdomen requires judgment and must take into consideration the patient's history, physical examination, and laboratory/radiologic testing.
- Keeping the differential diagnosis broad is prudent. Causes of acute abdomen may range from mechanical (e.g., bowel obstruction) to ischemic (e.g., superior mesenteric artery [SMA] thrombosis) to infectious (e.g., appendicitis), etc.

- The most common symptom indicating an acute abdomen is severe, intractable abdominal pain, attributed to peritoneal inflammation.
- Pertinent information: What is the duration of symptoms? What is the nature/quality of abdominal pain? What is the patient's relevant medical/surgical history? What are the vital signs?

Physical Examination

- Abdominal inspection, palpation, and percussion; note any surgical scars or hernias, particularly in the inguinal region.
- Some patients with significant peritoneal irritation will not tolerate sitting up in bed for posterior chest auscultation or rolling over for a rectal examination because of the severity of their abdominal pain.
- Rebound tenderness
  - Rebound tenderness is indicative of peritoneal inflammation. This is elicited by palpation of the abdomen with light pressure and observation of the patient's response as different areas of the abdomen are examined.
  - Rebound tenderness is present when the patient experiences pain instead of relief with the release of pressure on the abdomen.
  - Palpation should be done gently, since it can cause excruciating pain in the patient with peritonitis. Some consider aggressive assessment of rebound tenderness to be generally unnecessary and downright mean.
  - Pain with percussion on the anterior abdominal wall may be the most reliable test.
  - Tapping on the sole of a patient's foot can also transmit vibrations to the abdominal cavity, and patients with an acute abdomen will not be able to tolerate this without discomfort.
- Guarding (please don't touch my tummy)
  - Involuntary guarding is another frequent finding in an acute abdomen and signifies tonic muscle contraction secondary to irritation of the peritoneum.
  - To distinguish involuntary guarding from voluntary guarding, apply constant pressure to the abdominal wall in a location far away from the point of maximal pain, and ask the patient to take a deep breath and relax.
  - If the abdominal wall muscles remain contracted despite this, involuntary guarding is likely present. This differs from voluntary guarding, which is the voluntary contraction of the abdominal wall muscles in response to pain.
  - Rigidity of the abdominal wall muscles due to involuntary guarding is a highly significant clinical finding.

Clinical Pearls

- It is critical to perform ongoing assessment of the hemodynamic status of the patient with a suspected acute abdomen and to provide supportive care until surgical evaluation is completed.

- The administration of opioid analgesics may confound or blunt findings indicating significant abdominal pathology, although this generally does not result in incorrect treatment decisions. All other things being equal, stubbornly refusing to provide appropriate analgesics to provide some relief of pain is just cruel and unnecessary.

- Patients with an acute abdomen should undergo a biochemical assessment to include complete blood count (CBC) and basic metabolic panel (BMP), urinalysis (UA), and pregnancy test (for females of reproductive age). Imaging studies should be obtained on the basis of the clinical question to be answered (e.g., CT scan of the abdomen to evaluate for potential small bowel obstruction [SBO]). This workup should be performed quickly, and serial abdominal exams may be necessary over the course of several hours in a patient at risk for developing an acute abdomen.

HERNIA

- A hernia is a defect in an anatomic structure (most commonly the abdominal fascia), which permits protrusion of abdominal viscera.
- For the purposes of consultation on hospitalized patients, there are 3 main categories: reducible (no big whoop), incarcerated (big whoop), and strangulated (huge hairy deal).
    - A **reducible hernia** is one that can easily return through its fascial defect with gentle manipulation.
    - An **incarcerated hernia is one that is irreducible** (i.e., it is not possible to return viscera to the appropriate intra-abdominal location).
    - A **strangulated hernia** is an incarcerated hernia in which the blood flow to the hernia contents is compromised leading to ischemia and possible necrosis. Associated signs include pain, erythema of the overlying skin, leukocytosis, and fever. **A strangulated hernia is a surgical emergency.**
- Pertinent information: What is the location and duration of the hernia? Is there scar overlying hernia? What is the patient's surgical history? Are there associated symptoms? What is the status of the hernia (i.e., strangulated, incarcerated, or reducible)? Is there fever, leukocytosis, or erythema of the skin overlying the hernia?

- **Physical examination**: Diagnosis of a hernia is ideally made by examining the patient in a standing position with the patient performing the Valsalva maneuver or coughing. Many hospitalized patients may not be able to stand in which case having the patient perform a Valsalva maneuver while supine is appropriate. A mass that protrudes is a hernia until proven otherwise.
- **Treatment**
  - Gentle attempts at hernia reduction are appropriate.
  - To perform a basic reduction, place the patient supine in the Trendelenburg position and slowly apply firm, constant, circular pressure with the palm of the hand on the hernia.
  - Abdominal pain after hernia reduction should prompt suspicion of ischemic bowel, and a surgery consultation is appropriate.
  - Patients with hernias may be candidate for surgical repair. Therefore, a nonurgent surgery consult should be called even if the hernia is reduced (the consult can wait until morning).
  - Trusses or binders are usually not effective in the treatment of hernias.
- **Clinical pearls**: Hernias are classified by both anatomy and status. Over 75% of hernias occur in the inguinal region, 10% are incisional or ventral hernias, 3% are femoral, and the rest are unusual types. The location is of less concern than the status of the hernia. Not all incarcerated hernias are strangulated.

BOWEL OBSTRUCTION

- Bowel obstruction may represent an urgent condition requiring surgical intervention.
- The most common causes of obstruction differ between small versus large bowel, but it is critical to assess all patients with bowel obstruction for hemodynamic stability, to stop oral intake, and to start fluid resuscitation.

Small Bowel Obstruction

- The most common causes of SBO are adhesions from previous abdominal operations, incarcerated hernias, and cancer.
- Classic signs/symptoms of SBO include abdominal distension, nausea, vomiting, diffuse abdominal pain, and cessation of flatus and bowel movements.

- As soon as an SBO is diagnosed, the patient should be made NPO; IV fluids should be started at a maintenance rate; and a nasogastric tube (NGT) should be placed and connected to low intermittent wall suction (presuming the patient has significant distention, nausea, and/or emesis).

- Pertinent information: What is the duration of symptoms? Is there a history of bowel obstruction and how was it managed? When was the last bowel movement or passage of flatus? What are the vital signs? Is there a history of abdominal or pelvic operations?

- Basic laboratory testing should be performed to look for electrolyte or hematologic abnormalities.

- **Physical examination:** Note abdominal scars or hernias (e.g., umbilical, inguinal, incisional), any evidence of affected stool or rectal mass on rectal exam, output from the NGT, and urine output. **If peritoneal signs are present, there's badness in that belly and urgent surgical consultation is indicated!**

- **Diagnosis**
  - An obstructive series should be obtained. Critical findings include evidence of intra-abdominal free air (indicative of likely bowel perforation), air-fluid levels within the small bowel, and presence/absence of colonic or rectal air (more suggestive of ileus or partial obstruction rather than complete SBO).
  - A CT scan of the abdomen and pelvis is helpful to identify a transition point and signs of intestinal ischemia.

- **Treatment:** Patients with peritonitis or significant abdominal pain after NGT decompression may have ischemic bowel, and surgery should be called urgently! Nonsurgical management with **fluid resuscitation and NGT decompression is the standard initial treatment for SBO.**

Large Bowel Obstruction

- Often similar in presentation to SBO, large bowel obstruction (LBO) frequently results in symptoms of abdominal distention and crampy pain as well as nausea/emesis and loss of appetite.

- Common causes include colorectal cancer, volvulus (cecal or sigmoid), stricture (often from diverticular disease), fecal impaction, and colonic pseudo-obstruction (not true LBO).

- It may be difficult to differentiate between mechanical LBO and colonic pseudo-obstruction (i.e., Ogilvie syndrome), which results from colonic dysmotility and may be seen in a variety of clinical settings. Your grandmother was right, you can die from constipation.

- Pertinent information: What is the timing of onset of symptoms (acute vs. gradual)? Is there a history of constipation or changes in recent bowel movement frequency or stool character? What is the patient's medical/surgical history?
- **Diagnosis**
  - Imaging with plain abdominal films and/or CT scan of the abdomen and pelvis is necessary to distinguish between SBO and LBO.
  - Imaging findings of intra-abdominal free air, kidney bean appearance of the colon (suggestive of volvulus), or intramural air (concerning for bowel ischemia) may constitute surgical emergencies.
- **Treatment**
  - **Surgical consultation should be obtained in all cases of suspected LBO.**
  - Initial treatment with NGT decompression and fluid resuscitation is appropriate.
  - Similar to SBO, patients with peritonitis on abdominal exam generally require urgent surgical intervention.
  - Depending on the etiology of LBO, colonoscopic decompression or stenting may also be a possible treatment option.

APPENDICITIS

- Acute appendicitis is an urgent consultation, although IV antibiotics may help temporize prior to definitive management.
- Appendicitis results when obstruction of the appendiceal lumen (secondary to infections, fecaliths, lymphoid hyperplasia, neoplasm, etc.) causes appendiceal venous outflow obstruction and ultimately, appendiceal wall ischemia.
- The classic presentation involves periumbilical pain, which then localizes to the right lower quadrant (RLQ) and is associated with fever, nausea, and poor appetite.
- Pertinent information: Duration of symptoms and any progression of symptoms since onset. Is there any personal or family history of inflammatory bowel disease? Is there dysuria, hematuria, flank pain, or changes in bowel movements? For female patients, it is especially important to note gynecologic history to assess for ovarian cysts or torsion, sexually transmitted infections, etc.
- **Physical examination**
  - Vital signs (fever? tachycardia?)

- Abdominal exam: Apply gentle pressure, beginning farthest away from painful area. Note signs of guarding or rebound, and whether these findings are focal or diffuse. Check for accessory signs like Rovsing sign (RLQ pain evoked upon palpation of the left lower quadrant [LLQ]) or the psoas sign (RLQ pain with resisted right hip flexion while lying supine or right hip extension while lying on the left side).
- Check for costovertebral angle tenderness.
- A pelvic exam should be performed on all female patients.
- **Diagnosis**
  - Lab tests should include CBC and a UA.
  - CT scan is the diagnostic method of choice in adults, since it is rapid, sensitive, and specific for identifying appendicitis.
  - Abdominal ultrasound (US) is the initial imaging modality of choice in pediatric patients to help reduce radiation exposure.
  - In pregnant patients, abdominal MRI or US is frequently used to minimize radiation exposure.
- **Treatment**
  - Appendectomy is the conventional treatment for appendicitis in patients who are appropriate operative candidates.
  - An accumulating body of evidence supports a course of antibiotic therapy as an alternative to surgery.
  - Many patients require adjunctive treatment, such as percutaneous drainage of periappendiceal abscess.

ACUTE CHOLECYSTITIS

- This is generally an elective consultation.
- Acute cholecystitis is a syndrome of acute gallbladder inflammation, right upper quadrant (RUQ) pain, and leukocytosis that often occurs in the setting of cystic duct obstruction.
- Cystic duct obstruction is often caused by gallstones, but cholecystitis may occur without gallstones in critically ill patients and other clinical contexts, which is then called "acalculous cholecystitis."
- Pertinent information: Is the patient septic? Are there signs of gallstones obstructing the common duct (pancreatitis, high alkaline phosphatase and transaminases, common duct dilation)? Is there any history of biliary colic?
- **Physical examination**
  - Typical exam findings include RUQ or midepigastric pain and tenderness.

- Check for Murphy sign by palpating the RUQ while asking the patient to inspire. If the patient arrests the breath mid-inspiration or has severe pain, the Murphy sign is positive. Murphy sign may be falsely negative in the elderly, obese, or those who have received analgesics.
- Charcot triad is seen in ascending cholangitis and consists of fever, abdominal pain, and jaundice. Not to be outdone, Reynolds has a pentad (fever, abdominal pain, jaundice, hypotension, and mental status changes) for severe, suppurative cholangitis. You don't want either.

- **Diagnosis**
  - Obtain CBC, complete metabolic profile (CMP), and lipase.
  - RUQ US. Features of cholecystitis include gallbladder wall thickening or edema, a positive sonographic Murphy sign, and pericholecystic fluid. US may also show common bile duct dilation, indicating possible choledocholithiasis.
  - If the US is nondiagnostic, cholescintigraphy (e.g., HIDA scan) can identify cystic duct obstruction by edema or gallstones and may be helpful in making the diagnosis.

- **Treatment**
  - For acute cholecystitis, start appropriate antibiotic therapy with the aim to cover gastrointestinal (GI) flora including anaerobes and gram-negative rods.
  - **Laparoscopic cholecystectomy** is the conventional treatment for acute cholecystitis in patients who are appropriate surgical candidates.
  - In patients who are not appropriate surgical candidates, antibiotic therapy is appropriate.
  - For those who have symptom progression or fail to improve with antibiotics alone, drainage of the gallbladder is indicated. This is often accomplished by percutaneous cholecystostomy tube placement.
  - Related conditions include **gallstone pancreatitis, choledocholithiasis, and biliary sepsis.** Consider endoscopic retrograde cholangiopancreatography if there is ongoing common bile duct obstruction. Interval cholecystectomy is recommended after resolution of active inflammation as indicated by decreased abdominal pain and downtrending lipase, alkaline phosphatase, and transaminases.

PANCREATITIS

- Pancreatitis is an inflammatory process of the pancreas that is a common cause of abdominal pain and usually resolves with medical management alone.
- Gallstones and excess consumption of potent potables run neck and neck for the number one cause of acute pancreatitis.
- Common symptoms are severe epigastric abdominal pain that radiates to the back, nausea, and vomiting.
- Consult surgery for patients with severe or complicated pancreatitis. These patients can decline precipitously and may require prompt surgical intervention.
- **Diagnosis**
  - Lab tests including CBC, CMP, amylase, and lipase should be obtained.
  - Amylase and lipase greater than 3 times the normal upper limit is strongly suggestive of acute pancreatitis.
  - Imaging such as CT or MRI with IV contrast may help establish the diagnosis when it is uncertain.
  - Imaging is also useful for detecting necrosis and other local complications in patients who present with severe pancreatitis or sepsis or have clinical deterioration after initial presentation.
- **Treatment**
  - **Early aggressive fluid resuscitation** and close monitoring for signs of organ failure are critical.
  - Pain control with IV opiates is often necessary. Morphine is generally avoided because of the theoretical potential for increases in sphincter of Oddi pressure.
  - Patients should initially be kept NPO. Many patients may be able to resume oral nutrition in the first few days as symptoms and laboratory values improve.
  - Patients with moderate to severe pancreatitis may not be able to resume oral nutrition in the first 5 to 7 days. In these cases, enteral feeding with a nasojejunal tube is preferred. In patients who do not tolerate enteral feedings, total parenteral nutrition may be required.
  - Prophylactic antibiotics are not recommended in acute pancreatitis, although they are useful when extrapancreatic infection is suspected, and in infected pancreatic necrosis.

- **Complications**
  - Local complications include acute peripancreatic fluid collection, pseudocyst, acute necrotic collection, and walled-off necrosis.
  - These complications often respond to conservative treatment but may require drainage procedures if symptomatic.
  - **Infected necrosis** should be suspected in patients who have evidence of pancreatic necrosis on imaging and develop signs of sepsis or fail to improve after 7 to 10 days. This is an **urgent surgical problem!** Start appropriate antibiotics. Patients may require percutaneous drainage or surgical necrosectomy if antibiotic treatment alone fails.
  - Vascular complications include splanchnic venous thrombosis and pseudoaneurysm formation. These may require treatment with anticoagulation and embolism, respectively, based on the clinical scenario.
  - Abdominal compartment syndrome is a rare but significant complication of pancreatitis that may require urgent surgical decompression.
  - Systemic complications of pancreatitis include acute respiratory distress syndrome, acute tubular necrosis, and other manifestations of organ dysfunction.

DIVERTICULITIS

- Diverticulitis is defined as inflammation of colonic diverticula that can lead to complications including local infection, perforation, abscess, stricture, and fistula formation.
- This is usually an elective consultation but may become urgent or emergent if the patient develops free air or diffuse peritonitis.
- Generally, uncomplicated diverticulitis (i.e., minimal pain or derangement in laboratory values, and no perforation or abscess) may be treated in the outpatient setting with a liquid diet and 7 to 10 days of PO antibiotics that target GI flora.
- Complicated diverticulitis (i.e., with abscess, perforation, fistulization, or obstruction) requires inpatient treatment and warrants surgical consultation.
- Pertinent information: Are there signs of sepsis (e.g., fever, hypotension, tachycardia) or diffuse peritonitis? Is this the first episode of diverticulitis? Is the patient immunosuppressed? Has the patient failed outpatient treatment?

- **Physical examination**
  - Most patients will have localized tenderness to palpation, usually in the LLQ or suprapubic region.
  - Patients with diffuse tenderness to palpation require an urgent surgery consultation.
- **Diagnosis**
  - Obtain lab tests including a CBC and BMP.
  - CT abdomen and pelvis with IV contrast is the initial study of choice for stable patients.
- **Treatment**
  - The advantage of surgical consultation in this setting is 2-fold: to assist in management of the acute problem and to arrange follow-up of patients who may require elective colectomy after successful medical management of diverticulitis.
  - **The vast majority of patients do not require surgery in the acute setting** and will improve with medical management alone.
  - Many patients with pneumoperitoneum can be managed medically, although surgical consultation is recommended in this setting.
  - Most abscesses are adequately managed with percutaneous drain placement.
  - When surgery is required in the acute setting, usually a segmental colectomy is performed with an end colostomy to divert stool (i.e., Hartmann procedure).
  - Elective surgery is indicated in patients who are good surgical candidates with recurrent bouts of uncomplicated diverticulitis or one episode of complicated diverticulitis.
- **Complications**
  - For abscess formation, consult interventional radiology for consideration of percutaneous drainage. If the abscess is not drainable, treatment options include a course of antibiotics and surgical drainage.
  - Microperforation (or so-called contained perforation) is generally treated nonoperatively. If the patient clinically deteriorates, repeat imaging or surgical interventional may be needed.
  - **Perforation, obstruction, diffuse peritonitis, and sepsis require urgent surgical consultation.**

GASTROINTESTINAL BLEEDING

Most GI bleeds are managed medically with the assistance of therapeutic endoscopy, but these can become urgent or emergent surgery consultations.

Upper Gastrointestinal Bleeding

- Defined as bleeding in the GI tract proximal to the ligament of Treitz.
- The most common cause is peptic ulcer disease, and major risk factors include NSAID use and *Helicobacter pylori* infection.
- Other causes include variceal bleeding, esophagitis, gastritis, cancer, and Malory-Weiss tear.
- Hematemesis with red blood or coffee grounds is indicative of an upper GI bleed, as is melena (black tarry stool). Both tend to freak out the average patient.
- Pertinent information: Does the patient have a history of recurrent abdominal pain, reflux, dysphagia, or portal hypertension? Was the patient retching or coughing prior to hematemesis? Is the patient stable? What is their hematocrit? Is the patient taking anticoagulants or does he/she has a medical condition that may impair his/her hemostatic ability?
- **Physical examination**
  - Check for signs of volume depletion.
  - NG lavage often reveals blood or coffee ground–like material and can be helpful to clear the stomach for endoscopy.
  - Abdominal tenderness may or may not be present.
  - Look for melanotic stool on digital rectal exam and perform a stool guaiac test.
- **Treatment**
  - Resuscitation and correction of any coagulopathy should be top priority!
  - Ensure adequate IV access and prepare cross-matched blood if active bleeding is suspected.
  - **Endoscopy is first-line therapy in patients with upper GI bleeding.** It can be both diagnostic and therapeutic, and it may be repeated multiple times if bleeding recurs.
  - In patients who fail endoscopic management, surgery and/or interventional radiology should be considered for definitive control of bleeding.

Lower Gastrointestinal Bleeding

- Defined as bleeding distal to the ligament of Treitz.
- Hematochezia with maroon or red blood and/or passage of blood clots with stool is generally indicative of lower GI bleeding, although it may also be present when there is massive upper GI bleeding.
- Common causes include diverticular bleeding (most common), vascular malformations (common in elderly), neoplasms, colitis, ischemia, and inflammatory bowel disease.
- Generally, inflammatory causes of bleeding are associated with abdominal pain and diarrhea, while other causes are painless.
- Pertinent information: Does the patient have a history of recurrent abdominal pain, melena, diverticulosis, hemorrhoids, inflammatory bowel disease, or anal pathology? When was the patient's last colonoscopy and what did it show? Is the patient stable? What is their hematocrit?
- **Physical examination**
  - Check for signs of volume depletion.
  - **Don't skip the rectal exam!** Words to live by. Anal pathology such as hemorrhoids and anal fissures are common causes of blood in the stool or on toilet paper.
  - Is there any abdominal tenderness?
- **Treatment**
  - Similar to upper GI bleeding, resuscitation, correction of coagulopathy, adequate IV access, and preparation of cross-matched blood are critical, particularly if active bleeding is suspected.
  - Patients who have continued hemodynamic instability or suspected ongoing bleeding or cannot consume the colonoscopy preparation should undergo imaging to localize bleeding, usually CT angiography or radionuclide technetium-99m-labeled red-cell scintigraphy.
  - When bleeding is localized on imaging, angiography with embolization should be considered.
  - Patients who have hemodynamic stability and no signs of ongoing bleeding should undergo colon preparation and colonoscopy, which may be both diagnostic and therapeutic.
  - Rarely, bleeding is not able to be controlled with angiographic or endoscopic intervention. Surgical intervention should be considered in these cases.

MESENTERIC ISCHEMIA

- Acute mesenteric ischemia (AMI) is an emergency that can lead to bowel necrosis and death. It requires an **immediate surgical consultation!** There is a 60% to 80% mortality in patients with acute onset ischemia!

- Causes of AMI
    - Arterial embolism, usually to the SMA, is the most common cause of AMI, accounting for 40% to 50% of cases.
    - Arterial thrombosis is usually caused by thrombosis of a previously stenotic vessel. Less commonly it may be related to inflammation or dissection.
    - Mesenteric venous thrombosis leads to outflow obstruction and bowel edema. It is usually related to hypercoagulable state, trauma, or local inflammation.
    - Nonocclusive ischemia is due to impaired perfusion and vasoconstriction and is often related to low flow states such as heart failure, hypovolemia, and post–cardiac surgery.

- Chronic mesenteric ischemia (also called abdominal angina) is generally nonurgent and presents as abdominal pain after meals. More than 90% of cases are caused by progressive mesenteric atherosclerosis at the origins of vessels.

- Pertinent information: Does the patient have a history of postprandial abdominal pain? Was the onset of symptoms sudden? Is there a known source of emboli (e.g., atrial fibrillation, aortic plaque, endocarditis)? Is there a hypercoagulable state? Cancer? Any recent aortic instrumentation (such as cardiac catheterization)?

- **Physical examination**: Initially there are minimal physical findings (classically pain out of proportion to the exam) but as bowel ischemia and inflammation progress, the patient will develop abdominal distension, tenderness, and peritoneal signs. Watch for signs of sepsis and hypovolemia.

- **Diagnosis**
    - Check lab tests including CBC, CMP, lactic acid, and coagulation tests.
    - If stable, CT angiography of the abdomen and pelvis is the initial study of choice. Do not use PO contrast as this may obscure the mesenteric vessels.
    - If unstable, begin resuscitation and obtain abdominal plain films to look for free air or signs of bowel ischemia/necrosis.

- **Treatment**
  - Initial management includes IV fluid resuscitation, NG decompression, systemic anticoagulation to prevent thrombus propagation, and broad-spectrum IV antibiotics.
  - More definitive treatment is tailored to the cause of ischemia.
  - Embolic occlusion: Exploration with embolectomy is the definitive treatment. Mesenteric arteriography with thrombolysis may be considered in stable patients with no peritoneal signs.
  - Arterial thrombosis: Options include laparotomy with surgical revascularization and endovascular angioplasty and stenting.
  - Venous thrombosis: Anticoagulation alone is often effective. Laparotomy is required if there are signs of nonviable bowel.
  - Nonocclusive ischemia: Treatment of the underlying cause along with minimization of vasoconstrictors is important.
  - Patients with peritonitis require laparotomy to resect any necrotic bowel. All necrosis must go!

PERIANAL AND PERIRECTAL ABSCESS

- Nobody's favorite
- Generally, this is an elective consultation but may be urgent in the setting of sepsis or if the infectious process appears extensive.
- These abscesses usually form as a result of obstruction and infection of an anal crypt gland.
- Patients present with severe pain in the perianal area. Fever and malaise may also be present.
- Pertinent information: Are there the coexisting illnesses such as diabetes, a history of solid organ and bone marrow transplant, inflammatory bowel disease, radiation to the area, and a history of abscesses in this location?
- **Physical examination**
  - Findings include a fluctuant, very tender mass near the anus (yikes), often with erythema of the overlying skin.
  - Deeper abscesses may only be appreciated on a digital rectal exam.
  - How far does the erythema and induration extend? If the stigmata of infection spread rapidly and involve other perineal structures, then the patient may have **Fournier gangrene, which is a surgical emergency.** "Go, villain, fetch a surgeon."

- **Diagnosis**
  - Careful physical exam is critical, paying particular attention to the genitalia and perineum.
  - Imaging studies such as CT may be useful when a perirectal abscess is suspected but not palpable on exam.
- **Treatment**: Examination under anesthesia for abscess drainage is typically undertaken to manage perirectal abscesses.
- **Clinical pearls**
  - Many patients have a concomitant anal fistula and often require surgical fistulotomy at a later date.
  - Antibiotics alone may be effective for small or undrainable abscesses.
  - Fournier gangrene will necessitate wide debridement in the operating room with massive irrigation of the affected areas.

PNEUMOTHORAX

- Usually an urgent consultation but it can also be an emergent consultation if the patient is receiving positive pressure ventilation or if there is suspicion of a tension pneumothorax.
- Common symptoms include dyspnea and chest pain.
- Signs suggestive of **tension physiology** (e.g., tracheal deviation, distant or absent breath sounds on the affected side, hypotension, jugular venous distension) **should expedite intervention!**
- Pertinent information: What was the onset of the symptoms? Any new supplemental oxygen requirement? Possible etiologies (e.g., trauma, known blebs, positive pressure ventilation, recent procedures such as central line or pacemaker insertion)? Any available chest imaging?
- **Physical examination**
  - Overall clinical appearance including tachypnea, accessory respiratory muscle use, or difficulty speaking in full sentences.
  - Note if the patient has recently been or is currently on positive pressure ventilation. Always be wary of signs concerning for a tension pneumothorax.
- **Diagnosis**
  - **If a tension pneumothorax is suspected from history and clinical exam, no further diagnostic tests should be pursued, and treatment should be immediate!**

- If a simple pneumothorax is more likely and vital signs are stable, an erect chest radiograph (CXR) should be obtained urgently.
- Critical CXR findings include a visceral pleural line and peripheral radiolucency (showing air in the peripheral chest with a lack of lung markings). A deep sulcus sign may also be present on a supine film with displacement of the costophrenic angle inferiorly.

- **Treatment**
  - Tension pneumothorax: Immediately place a large-bore (14G or 16G) angiocatheter in the second interspace above the rib at the midclavicular line of the affected side, followed by a pleasing hissing sound and patient improvement. A chest tube should subsequently be placed on that side.
  - Simple pneumothorax: Most will require open tube thoracostomy or percutaneous tube thoracostomy. Expectant management with serial chest radiographs may suffice in a young, asymptomatic patient with a small pneumothorax (up to 15%) who is not on positive pressure ventilation.

NECROTIZING SOFT TISSUE INFECTIONS

- Necrotizing soft tissues infections (NSTIs) include necrotizing cellulitis, myositis, and fasciitis, which may lead to tissue necrosis and systemic sepsis. NSTIs have high mortality rates, which makes it critical to initiate treatment as soon as possible.
- **Early detection and surgical debridement are the keys to reducing morbidity and mortality! Call surgery when NSTI is suspected.** Again, all necrosis must go.
- Risk factors include diabetes, immune compromise, peripheral vascular disease, recent surgery, trauma, or break in skin integrity.
- Causative organisms
  - Type I: polymicrobial, usually anaerobic organisms in addition to *Enterobacter* and *Streptococcus* spp.
  - Type II: monomicrobial, usually group A streptococcus or other β-hemolytic streptococci may be associated with toxic shock syndrome.
- Necrotizing fasciitis spreads rapidly and insidiously along fascial planes, sparing the overlying tissue. **Skin findings occur late, only after significant spread of infection!**

- Pertinent information: Does the patient have risk factors for NSTI? What is the time course of symptoms? Are symptoms progressing or is the patient's clinical status deteriorating despite antibiotic treatment? Does the patient have pain out of proportion to exam findings? Was there an inciting event?
- **Physical examination**
  - Skin findings may progress from normal, to erythema and induration, to color changes with blue/black spots, bullae, crepitus, and frank necrosis.
  - **Pain out of proportion to exam findings is a key warning sign for all NSTIs!**
  - There may be fluid discharge from the wound, classically grayish and thin ("dishwater fluid").
  - Signs of systemic toxicity such as fever, leukocytosis, and tachycardia may be present with advanced infections, but these may not appear until late in the disease course.
- **Treatment**
  - **Wide surgical debridement, antibiotics, and supportive care constitute definitive treatment for NSTIs!**
  - Consult surgery immediately if there is clinical concern for NSTI.
  - Early debridement is essential!
  - Concurrent broad-spectrum antibiotic treatment is recommended and generally includes clindamycin (for antitoxin effects) as well as an agent active against methicillin-resistant *Staphylococcus aureus* (MRSA).

ISCHEMIC LOWER EXTREMITY

- Now let's not lose our legs over this.
- An acutely ischemic extremity is an emergency. **Call a vascular surgery consult immediately!** Time is leg.
- Symptoms of acute arterial insufficiency can occur abruptly, although collateral flow may temporize the severity.
- Limb ischemia may be due to acute events (embolic disease) or chronic disease (atherosclerosis). **Acute ischemia is an emergency because perfusion must be reestablished as soon as possible (preferably within 6 h) to achieve limb salvage.** Unlike patients with chronic disease, many patients with acute

obstruction have not developed collateral circulation to supply the lower leg.

- Phlegmasia cerulea dolens (PCD, say that three times fast) is a rare cause of extremity ischemia due to massive acute deep venous thrombosis that leads to pain, swelling, cyanosis, and edema that impair arterial flow.
- **In any situation where acute limb ischemia is suspected, do not hesitate to call a surgical consult.**
- Pertinent information: What is the suspected source? Embolism (atrial fibrillation/arrhythmia, left ventricular aneurysm, abdominal aortic aneurysm, or popliteal aneurysm)? Chronic atherosclerotic disease? Did the pain come on suddenly? Is the pain unilateral? Has this patient had any endovascular therapy or vascular surgery? If so, what interventions have been performed? Where does the bypass start and end?
- **Physical examination**
  - On examination, look for the 6 P's: pain, pallor, pulselessness, paresthesias, paralysis, and poikilothermia (a highfalutin word that starts with a P for coolness).
  - Status of collateral flow: Perform a Doppler examination in the femoral, popliteal, dorsalis pedis (DP), and posterior tibial (PT) arteries. Be able to tell the consultant if there is a temperature difference in the extremities and at what level (foot, shin, thigh, or whole leg).
  - Severity of ischemia: The peripheral nerve is the tissue that is most sensitive to ischemia. The most sensitive test to determine if the foot is viable is to test for proprioception of the toes. This will diminish within 5 minutes of cessation of blood flow. Next, test motor function and light touch.
  - In patients with PCD, exam findings include edema and tenderness that can progress to cyanosis with bullae formation and compartment syndrome.
- **Treatment**
  - Most patients are started on intravenous heparin therapy.
  - Possible interventions for arterial ischemia include surgical bypass, endovascular angioplasty and stenting, thrombectomy, or locally delivered intravascular thrombolytics.
  - Patients with PCD may require thrombectomy or thrombolysis.
  - Indications for subsequent treatment with anticoagulation or antiplatelet agents vary depending on the cause of ischemia.

ISCHEMIC ULCER OF THE LOWER EXTREMITY

- Ischemic ulcer of the lower extremity is an elective consultation.
- Pertinent information: What is the location of the ulcer? Has this patient had vascular surgery? If so, where does the bypass start and end? Where are the scars? Is the patient a diabetic? Are blood glucose levels well controlled? Are they ever?
- Ischemic ulcers are commonly found on the first metatarsal head or tips of the toes and are due to a combination of unrecognized trauma, poor circulation, and infection. They are distinguished from venous stasis ulcers by location (usually found near the medial malleolus), appearance (heaped up, engorged edges), and pain.
- Diabetes can cause calcified vessels that make ankle-brachial indices unreliable. Some diabetics develop ulcers secondary to microvascular disease without obvious atherosclerosis in the larger vessels.
- **Physical examination**
  - Palpate or perform a Doppler examination of the pulses in the femoral, popliteal, DP, and PT arteries.
  - Look for signs of infection (e.g., erythema, pain, fluctuance, purulent discharge with palpation).
  - Note the location of the ulcer, as this may give clues to the etiology.
  - Note the level of tissue that is exposed (i.e., bone, subcutaneous tissue, fascia, tendon).
- **Diagnosis**
  - Plain radiographs should be obtained to document osteomyelitis of the underlying bone. Any exposed bone is assumed to have osteomyelitis until proven otherwise.
  - Lower extremity segmental pressures mapping is a noninvasive method of quantifying arterial insufficiency.
- **Treatment**: Debridement or revascularization may be required.

PRESSURE ULCERS

- Pressure ulcers result from prolonged pressure to soft tissue over bony prominences.
- They most commonly occur in immobile patients over the occiput, sacrum, greater trochanter, and heels.
- Muscle and fat are more sensitive to pressure than skin or bone; thus patients with a small area of skin breakdown may have large areas of associated soft tissue necrosis.

- Pertinent information: Is the patient septic? Is the patient immobile? What is the extent and etiology of the patient's immobility? What is their current wound care management? Yes doctor, but was it present on admission?
- **Physical examination**
  - Note the location of the ulcer and whether there is necrotic tissue at its base or edges.
  - Stage the ulcer according to the National Pressure Ulcer Advisory Panel staging system:[1]
    - Stage 1: nonblanchable erythema of intact skin
    - Stage 2: partial-thickness skin loss with exposed dermis
    - Stage 3: full-thickness skin loss (in which fat and granulation tissue are often exposed)
    - Stage 4: full-thickness skin and tissue loss with exposed or directly palpable fascia, muscle, tendon, ligament, cartilage or bone in the ulcer (yuck)
    - Unstageable: full-thickness skin and tissue loss in which the extent of tissue damage cannot be confirmed because it is obscured by slough or eschar
- **Treatment**
  - A consult to a wound care specialist should be placed for first-line therapy of pressure ulcers unless there is concern that an ulcer is a source of sepsis or has a large amount of necrotic tissue that will require debridement.
  - Most superficial pressure ulcers heal (stage 1) with pressure off-loading and supportive care. Deeper ulcers (stage 2 and greater) in addition typically require more aggressive wound care.
  - Local wound care and optimization of nutrition are key for ulcer healing. Urinary and fecal continence needs to be maintained to prevent maceration and skin breakdown as well as contamination of the ulcer base.

References

1. Edsberg LE, Black JM, Goldberg M, et al. Revised national pressure ulcer advisory panel pressure injury staging system: revised pressure injury staging system. *J Wound Ostomy Continence Nurs* 2016;43:585-97.

Critical Care

29

David Pham and Adam Anderson

KEYS TO INTENSIVE CARE UNIT SURVIVAL

- Each hospital is different and each intensive care unit (ICU) within a hospital has its different habits. Everyone thinks he/she does it the right way, and this is our right way.
- **There are no inappropriate questions!** If you have something you want to know more about or have a problem, do not hesitate to ask. It is a team effort in the ICU, and a part of the duties of the residents, fellows, and attendings is to teach.
- ICU patients are very complex. Always try to divide and conquer. Stabilize the patient and then go from there. Think of the ABC's (airway, breathing, and circulation).
- **Know what resources are available to you and how to use them effectively! Your residents and co-interns should tell you how it really is.**
- The nurses, respiratory therapists, pharmacists, patient care technicians, and unit secretaries know what they're doing. This might be a rotation for you, but this is what they do day in and day out. They have useful insight and are valuable resources; listen to their input and concerns.
- Treat the patient and not the numbers. If something doesn't make sense, examine the patient again. You may find that something was overlooked.
- There is no "set it and forget it" in the ICU. Patients change rapidly in the ICU and part of excelling is being flexible and adapting to the dynamic situations.
- Thorough documentation is vital to patient care in the ICU. A basic ICU note should include admit date, length of stay, principle diagnosis, medications with drip rates, antibiotics with planned duration, ins and outs (I/Os), external devices and lines, ventilator settings, and code status.

LIFE IN THE INTENSIVE CARE UNIT

- The ICU can be chaotic and overwhelming with sick patients needing care acutely. This usually comes in waves rather than a steady stream. A good strategy is to develop a routine (or adopt someone else's) to make the most of your time and to ensure orders and tasks are being completed.
- Attention to detail makes a difference more so in the ICU than anywhere else. Being organized and having a plan will prepare you for success.
- Workflow is dependent on the hospital and ICU, but there are always significant differences between the day and night.
- To that end, this is a possible day and night routine in our ICU.

Daytime

- Receive updates of major events from your co-interns, nursing, and respiratory therapy upon arrival to the unit.
- Preround on your old patients with a chart review and physical examination. Know significant events from the last 24 hours that need to be discussed during rounds with the attending.
- Rounds are dependent on attending preference. Be prepared to discuss every aspect of the patient's history, problems, and plan.
- Go in the room with the attending to observe his/her exam and methodical approach.
- Enter orders for your colleagues during rounds. Call consultants either during rounds (if acceptable with the attending) or immediately after.
- Update sign-out and ICU boards throughout rounds with tasks.
- Daily notes should reflect what was discussed during rounds and also be a place to track antibiotics days, location and duration of central line, settings days on ventilator, deep venous thrombosis and stress ulcer prophylaxis, and code status.
- Throughout the day, it is imperative to evaluate the patients again and verify tasks are completed for the day. If consultants were called, confirm patients were evaluated and follow up on recommendations.
- Transfers out of the ICU can occur anytime depending on bed availability. A thorough transfer note and verbal sign-out helps transition care throughout the hospital.
- "Run the list" several times a day with the resident and fellow. They can help with tasks and can help explain why decisions were made.

Nighttime

- Hopefully, most daytime goals have been completed. Regardless, at the start of the shift, go through the checklist and verify what has been completed and what still needs to be finished.

- Getting accurate and pertinent sign-out from the day team will be vital if there is a shift change. Rounding at the bedside during handoff helps. Pending lab tests and patients who required a lot of active care during the day should be emphasized.

- Social and family issues are best conveyed with verbal sign-out.

- Several ICU admissions occur at night. This can make it difficult to follow up on goals that were discussed the day, again stressing the necessity of efficiency.

- Round again throughout the night to verify I/O goals are met; replete electrolytes and blood products. Patients commonly require additional diuretics to achieve goal fluid balance.

VENTILATORS

Suggestions for Initial Ventilator Settings
Basic Settings

- Mode
  - Assist control/volume control (AC/VC): Rate and tidal volume are set. Should "guarantee" a minimal minute ventilation and often the mode to start. Airway pressures are dependent on compliance.
  - Pressure-controlled (PC) ventilation: Rate and drive pressure are set. Tidal volume and minute ventilation are not "guaranteed" and depend on compliance.
  - Pressure-regulated volume control (AC/VC+ or PRVC): A mix of both VC and PC. Rate, target tidal volume, and inspiratory time are set. Understand VC and PC before trying to get PRVC.
  - Synchronous intermittent mandatory ventilation with pressure support ventilation (SIMV + PSV): Similar to AC except patient-triggered breaths are delivered with pressure support instead of full tidal volume.

- Tidal volume: Depends! Every patient is different but 6 mL/kg of ideal body weight for lung protective ventilation in acute respiratory distress syndrome patients. May need much, more or less depending on etiology of respiratory failure.

- Rate: Depends! Try to at least match the minute ventilation prior to intubation. Paralyzed patients will be set rate dependent, whereas nonparalyzed can overbreathe. Try to set backup rate a few below the patient's actual rate to avoid hyperventilation.
- FiO_2: Depends! 1.00, then titrate down (goal to get FiO_2 to ≤0.60 as quickly as possible).
- Positive end-expiratory pressure (PEEP): Depends! Obese or markedly hypoxemic patients will need more. Otherwise, start at 5 cm H_2O (monitor for auto-PEEP, especially with obstructive lung disease).

Advanced Settings
- Ask for help before you change these.
- Inspiratory flow: 50 to 60 L/min. With obstructive lung disease may need >100 L/min.
- Inspiration to expiration (I:E) ratio or inspiratory time: 1:2 to 1:3. This must be set with PCV and AC/VC+ (PRVC).
- Peak and plateau pressures: goal plateau pressure <30 cm H_2O; prefer peak pressure <45 cm H_2O.

Ventilator Adjustments

- PaO_2 of 60 mm Hg or greater is generally sufficient. Oxygenation is most affected by mean airway pressure. Adjustments to FiO_2, PEEP and I:E ratio can help increase oxygenation. Remember that the **oxygen saturations (SpO_2) and PaO_2 can be discordant**; sometimes it is necessary to verify that they correlate with an arterial blood gas.
- $PaCO_2$ is regulated by minute ventilation. Increasing the respiratory rate or tidal volume increases minute ventilation and decreases PCO_2.
- See Table 29-1 for suggested adjustments.

Trouble Shooting the Ventilator: Common Alarms

- Remember the ventilator is an active intervention in a patient's care. Managing ventilated patients require dynamic assessment of the patients' conditions, their goals, and working closely with the nurses and respiratory therapist who spend more of their time at the bedside of the patient.
- **Don't panic and approach the problem with a stepwise manner.**
- **Examine the patient** and evaluate the machine.

TABLE 29-1	SUGGESTIONS FOR VENTILATOR MANAGEMENT BASED ON PCO_2 AND PO_2[a]	
	PCO_2	PO_2
High	↑ tidal volume ↑ respiratory rate	↓ FiO_2
Low	↓ tidal volume ↓ respiratory rate	↑ FiO_2 ↑ PEEP

[a]Very general recommendations; must be individualized for each patient.

- Is there a patient problem? Is there a ventilator problem?
- Listen to the patient and observe them breathing on the ventilator.
- Recheck the ventilator settings.

High Pressure

- By far, the most common alarm you will encounter.
- Remember that high pressure means that the ventilator is encountering higher resistance as it attempts to pump air into the patient's lungs.
- Patient: Biting the tube (too awake)? Coughing (very common)? Mucous plug/increased secretions? Less lung compliance (increased pulmonary edema or pneumothorax)?
- Order a chest radiograph. What are the patient's vital signs?
- Machine: Obstructed endotracheal tube? Incorrect settings? Breath stacking? Examine the machine.
- If still having issues, **manually bag the patient** to eliminate the machine and continue to troubleshoot.

Low Pressure
Usually due to disconnected tubing or air leak in the circuit. Troubleshoot as mentioned in High Pressure section.

High Respiratory Rate

- Patient: pain or anxious (too awake)?
- Machine: autotriggering usually due to water in the tubing or kinking in tubing

Apnea
- Patient: Oversedated? Neurologic catastrophe?
- Machine: usually disconnected tubing

Oxygenation
- The knee-jerk impulse is to increase the FiO_2. **Don't panic!**
- Patient: Worsening of underlying disease? Dyssynchrony (more sedation)? Loss of PEEP? Too many secretions (suction)? Increased pulmonary edema (diuresis)?
- Machine: Wrong settings? Wrong mode (more synchrony with patient)?

Weaning Parameters

The method of weaning is not as relevant as knowing the appropriate time to wean. See Table 29-2.[1]

TABLE 29-2	GUIDELINES FOR ASSESSING WITHDRAWAL OF MECHANICAL VENTILATION

Patient's mental status: awake, alert, cooperative
PO_2 >60 mm Hg with an FiO_2 <0.5
PEEP ≤5 cm H_2O
PCO_2 and pH acceptable
Spontaneous tidal volume >5 mL/kg
Vital capacity >10 mL/kg
Minute ventilation <10 L/min
Maximum voluntary ventilation double of minute ventilation
Maximum negative inspiratory pressure ≥25 cm H_2O
Respiratory rate <30 breaths/min
Static compliance >30 mL/cm H_2O
Rapid shallow breathing index <100 breaths/L[a]
Stable vital signs following 30 min to 1 h spontaneous breathing trial

[a]Rapid shallow breathing index = respiratory rate/tidal volume in liters.
From Kollef MH, Micek ST. Critical Care. In: Foster C, Mistry NF, Peddi PF, Sharma S, eds. Washington Manual of Medical Therapeutics. 33rd ed. Philadelphia, PA: Lippincott Williams & Wilkins, 2010.

INTENSIVE CARE UNIT SEDATION/PARALYSIS

- Take a "PAD" approach (pain, agitation, delirium).
- Ventilated patients generally require analgesia. This is usually achieved through bolus or continuous IV infusion of opioids. See Table 29-3.[2]
- Achieve the desired level of analgesia/sedation with boluses before starting a continuous infusion. Specify the desired level of sedation (Table 29-4).[3] If the patient becomes uncomfortable, bolus to desired level of analgesia/sedation and then make small incremental changes in the drip rate.
- Titrate to minimum effective dose and **reassess the need for continuous drips daily.**
- Consider adding paralytics (Table 29-5)[3] for patients with very poor oxygenation or if patient-ventilator dyssynchrony persists despite adequate sedation causing difficulty with ventilation. **Ensure the patient is adequately sedated before adding paralytics.**
- The degree of paralysis is usually monitored by peripheral nerve stimulation and the train-of-four method. Complete paralysis is unnecessary for many patients.
- **Paralysis should be discontinued daily to determine the continued need for paralysis and to assess for adequate sedation.**

TABLE 29-3	RICHMOND AGITATION AND SEDATION SCALE
+4	Overtly combative, violent, immediate danger to staff
+3	Pulls or removes tubes or catheters; aggressive
+2	Frequent nonpurposeful movement, fights ventilator
+1	Anxious but movements not aggressive or vigorous
0	Alert and calm
−1	Not fully alert, but has sustained awakening (eye opening/eye contact) to voice ≥10 s
−2	Briefly awakens with <10 s eye contact to voice
−3	Movement or eye opening to voice (no eye contact)
−4	No response to voice, movement or eye opening to physical stimulation
−5	No response to voice or physical stimulation

Adapted from Ely EW, Truman B, Shintani A, et al. Monitoring sedation status over time in ICU patients: reliability and validity of the Richmond Agitation-Sedation Scale (RASS). JAMA 2003;289:2983-91, with permission.

TABLE 29-4	ICU SEDATION						
Drug	Bolus Dosing	Onset (Single Dose)	Duration (Single Dose)	Continuous Dilution	Maintenance Dose	Titration Increment	Comments
Fentanyl	25-100 µg, max 300 µg/ 15 min	1-2 min, peak 2-5 min	30-60 min	2500 µg/50 mL	50-200 µg/h	50 µg/h	Possible bradycardia with bolus doses[a]
Morphine	10-15 mg	5-10 min, peak 20 min	3-4 h	100 mg/100 mL	1-50 mg/h	2-5 mg/h	Possible hypotension due to histamine release[a]
Lorazepam	2-4 mg	20-40 min	3-6 h	40 mg/40 mL	0.5-4 mg/h	0.25 mg/h	Associated with acute tubular necrosis, lactic acidosis, and hyperosmolar states with prolonged infusion[a]
Midazolam	1-5 mg, max 15 mg in 15 min	1-4 min	30-60 min	50 mg/50 mL	1-8 mg/h	1 mg/h	Possible hypotension with bolus doses[a]

Propofol	Not recommended	1-2 min	30 min	1000 mg/100 mL	25-50 µg/kg per minute	10 µg/kg per minute	10% lipid = 1.1 kcal/mL; possible hypotension, bradycardia, hypertriglyceridemia, pancreatitis, and propofol-related infusion syndrome
Dexmedetomidine	Not recommended	10 min	30 min	400 µg/100 mL	0.2-0.7 µg/kg per hour	0.1 µg/kg per hour	Possible hypotension, bradycardia; doses up to 1.5 µg/kg per hour have been safely used for up to 30 d

aProlonged effect in renal and hepatic failure.
Adapted from Casabar E, Portell J, eds. Tool Book: Drug Dosing and Usage Guideline. 10th ed. St. Louis, MO: Department of Pharmacy, Barnes-Jewish Hospital, Washington University Medical Center, 2012.

TABLE 29-5	NEUROMUSCULAR BLOCKING AGENTS						
Drug	Bolus Dosing (mg/kg)	Onset (Single Dose)	Duration (Single Dose)	Continuous Dilution	Maintenance Dose Range (μg/kg per minute)	Titration Increment (μg/kg per minute)	Comments
Pancuronium	0.05-0.1	2-4 min	90-100 min	50 mg/50 mL	1-2	0.25	May cause mild tachycardia; effects prolonged in renal and hepatic failure
Vecuronium	0.05-0.1	2-4 min	35-45 min	50 mg/100 mL	0.5-1.5	0.25	Effects prolonged in renal and hepatic failure
Atracurium	0.3-0.5	2-3 min	25-35 min	500 mg/100 mL	5-25	5	May cause histamine release; dose may escalate over time. Metabolized by Hoffmann elimination

| Rocuronium | 0.6-1 | 1-2 min | 30 min | 200 mg/200 mL | 8-12 | 0.8-1.2 | Effects prolonged in renal and hepatic failure |
| Cisatracurium | 0.1-0.2 | 2-3 min | 45-60 min | 200 mg/100 mL | 2-10 | 2 | Metabolized by Hoffmann elimination |

Adapted from Casabar E, Portell J, eds. Tool Book: Drug Dosing and Usage Guidelines. 10th ed. St. Louis, MO: Department of Pharmacy, Barnes-Jewish Hospital, Washington University Medical Center, 2012.

SHOCK

Hemodynamic Profiles Associated With Shock

The hemodynamic parameters associated with the major forms of shock are presented in Table 29-6.

Treatment of Shock

- **Determine the type of shock first! Management depends on etiology. Not everyone needs IV fluids.**
- **Fluid resuscitation** is vital for distributive and hypovolemic shock. Crystalloid (normal saline or lactated Ringer's) should be started immediately. For hemorrhagic shock, blood products should be administered.
- Use of **vasopressors and/or inotropes** may be necessary. Vasopressors are generally titrated to a mean arterial pressure of ≥60 mm Hg. Afterload reduction and inotropes may be needed in cardiogenic shock. See Table 29-7 for dosages.[4]

DRIPS

Other intravenous drips commonly used in the ICU are presented in Table 29-7.[4]

SUGGESTIONS FOR PROPHYLAXIS

- For venous thromboembolic and gastrointestinal prophylaxis, see Chapter 7, Admissions.
- Decubitus ulcers: turning patient several times a day, vigilant skin care, egg crate mattress, flotation bed, and ensuring adequate nutrition
- Deconditioning: physical therapy, occupational therapy, and nutritional support
- Aspiration precautions: Elevate head of the bed >30° and provide adequate suctioning.
- Infection: Maintain oral hygiene; keep track of all lines (peripheral IV, central line, arterial lines, nasogastric tube, feeding tubes, Foley catheters) and remove as soon as no longer needed. Target or discontinue antibiotic therapy per guidelines to reduce induction of resistance and development of *Clostridium difficile* colitis.
- Follow isolation (respiratory or contact) precautions at all times and practice scrupulous hand hygiene.

TABLE 29-6 HEMODYNAMIC PROFILES ASSOCIATED WITH SHOCK

	Extremities	CVP	CI/CO	SVR	SvO_2	PCWP
Hypovolemic (hemorrhagic)	Cool	↓	↓	↑	↓	↓
Cardiogenic (MI, CHF, tamponade)	Cool	↑	↓	↑	↓	↑
Distributive (septic, pancreatitis)	Warm	↓	↑	↓	N to ↑	N to ↓

CVP, central venous pressure; CI, cardiac index; CO, cardiac output; SVR, systemic vascular resistance; SvO_2, mixed venous oxygen saturation; PCWP, pulmonary capillary wedge pressure; MI, myocardial infarction; CHF, congestive heart failure; N, normal; ↓, decreased; ↑, increased.

TABLE 29-7	COMMONLY USED INTENSIVE CARE UNIT DRIPS		
	Receptor Activity	Dosage	Comments
Vasopressors			
Dopamine	α, β, dopamine	1-3 µg per minute for renal and splanch-nic (dopamine)	Dose-dependent activation
		3-10 µg/kg/min for increase in cardiac con-tractility (β)	
		10 µg/kg per minute for vasoconstriction (α)	
Epinephrine	α, β	Start at: 0.1 µg/kg per minute	Drug of choice for anaphylactic shock
		Titrate: to MAP ≥60 mm Hg	Potent vasoconstrictor
Norepinephrine	α, β	Start at: 0.01 µg/kg per minute	Vasoconstrictor
		Titrate: to MAP ≥60 mm Hg	
Vasopressin	V1a, V1b, V2	Hypotension/shock: 0.04 units/min, do not titrate	
		GI bleed: 0.4 units/min	
Dobutamine	α, β	Start at: 2.5 µg/kg per minute	Has inotropic and chronotropic properties, causes reflex peripheral vasodilation
		Titrate: to desired effect	
		Usual max dose: 20 µg/kg per minute	
Milrinone	PDE III inhibitor resulting in reduced degradation of cAMP and in increased calcium influx	Loading dose: 50 µg/kg over 10 min	Inotrope, direct peripheral vasodilator
		Maintenance dose: 0.25-0.75 µg/kg per minute	Decrease dose in renal dysfunction.

Vasodilators/Afterload Reducers

Clevidipine	Dihydropyridine calcium channel blocker is highly selective for vascular smooth muscle resulting in a decrease of SVR	Start: 1-2 mg/h Titrate: Double dose every 90 s, can reduce increase as approaches target BP	Do not exceed 1000 mL/24 h due to lipid load, formulated in 20% fat emulsion. No decrease in CO or contractility.
Nitroglycerine	Converted to NO that activates guanylyl cyclase resulting in cGMP production that causes vascular smooth muscle relaxation	Start at: 5-10 µg/min Titrate: 10-20 µg/min every 5 min until desired effect	Tachyphylaxis can occur. At high doses, reflex tachycardia can occur.
Nitroprusside	Same as nitroglycerine	Start at: 0.3-0.5 µg/kg per minute Titrate: to desired effect Usual max dose: 10 µg/kg per minute	Signs of toxicity include metabolic acidosis, tremors, seizures, and coma. Check sodium thiocyanate levels with prolonged use. Do not use in renal failure.

MAP, mean arterial pressure; GI, gastrointestinal; PDE III, phosphodiesterase; BP, blood pressure; SVR, systemic vascular resistance.
Adapted from Casabar E, Portell J, eds. Tool Book: Drug Dosing and Usage Guidelines. 15th ed. St. Louis, MO: Department of Pharmacy, Barnes-Jewish Hospital, Washington University Medical Center, 2016.

References

1. Kollef MH, Micek ST. Critical Care. In: Foster C, Mistry NF, Peddi PF, Sharma S, eds. *Washington Manual of Medical Therapeutics*. 33rd ed. Philadelphia, PA: Lippincott Williams & Wilkins, 2010.

2. Ely EW, Truman B, Shintani A, et al. Monitoring sedation status over time in ICU patients: reliability and validity of the Richmond Agitation-Sedation Scale (RASS). *JAMA* 2003;289:2983-91.

3. Casabar E, Portell J, eds. *Tool Book: Drug Dosing and Usage Guideline*. 10th ed. St. Louis, MO: Department of Pharmacy, Barnes-Jewish Hospital, Washington University Medical Center, 2012.

4. Casabar E, Portell J, eds. *Tool Book: Drug Dosing and Usage Guidelines*. 15th ed. St. Louis, MO: Department of Pharmacy, Barnes-Jewish Hospital, Washington University Medical Center, 2016.

Guide to Procedures

30

Matthew Freer

VASCULAR ACCESS

Ultrasound-Guided Central Venous Access

- The use of ultrasound guidance for the placement of internal jugular (IJ) central venous catheters is superior to the landmark-guided technique because of an improvement in average access time, reduction in number of attempts, improved success rate, and possibly decreased complication rate. Ultrasound guidance may also be used for subclavian and femoral venous access, although the benefit for these procedures is less clear.

- **Indirect guidance** refers to assessing the vascular structures using 2D ultrasound prior to performing needle puncture and venous canalization.

- **Direct guidance** refers to the use of real-time ultrasound images during the needle puncture. The view can be either transverse (a cross section of the vein) or longitudinal (visualizing the vein on its long access). The transverse technique, which has been shown to be easier to learn by inexperienced physicians, will be described here.

- It is possible to distinguish veins from arteries using ultrasound.

  - Veins, in contrast to arteries, are more easily compressible with application of anterior-posterior pressure with the ultrasound probe. Central veins tend to be larger and less circular than adjacent arteries, but this can be misleading (e.g., in patients with low intravascular volume).

  - The relationship of the vein to the artery can also be useful: The IJ is typically anterolateral to the carotid artery. The femoral vein is typically medial to the femoral artery.

  - Doppler ultrasonography with color flow can help identify arteries on the basis of pulsatile flow, but this can be misleading as well (e.g., in patients with severe tricuspid regurgitation).

- See Table 30-1 for all you need to know about vascular access.

TABLE 30-1 ALL YOU REALLY NEED TO KNOW ABOUT VASCULAR ACCESS

Type	Description	Common Uses	Duration of Use
Triple-lumen catheter	Three separate lumens Placed via the Seldinger technique usually at the bedside Subclavian or internal jugular veins preferred, femoral vein can be used	When peripheral access is exhausted and in emergency situations Blood may be drawn from the catheter.	Short- to intermediate-term use (days to weeks) There is no need to routinely replace lines unless infection is suspected, and lines should never be changed over a guidewire. Replace femoral lines more frequently, although recent studies suggest that infection rates with femoral lines are lower than previously thought.
Hickman catheter	Placed by surgery or interventional radiology (single- or multilumen) Subcutaneously tunneled Dacron cuff at the skin entry site Located in subclavian or internal jugular vein (tip is located near the right atrium)	Long-term intravenous medications and/or fluids Blood may be drawn from the catheter.	Long-term use May be left in place indefinitely as long as functioning properly. Must be removed by surgery or radiology.

Hohn catheter	Single- or double-lumen catheters Placed via Seldinger technique (usually by interventional radiology) without a subcutaneous tunnel "Power" Hohn can be used to inject contrast quickly (e.g., for PE-protocol CT).	Placed when peripheral access is exhausted or longer-term outpatient access is needed. Administration of medications and fluids Blood may be drawn from the catheter.	Intermediate-term use (up to 6 wk) May be removed at the bedside (same as a triple-lumen catheter).
Implanted venous access device (Port-A-Cath)	Placed subcutaneously by a surgeon or interventional radiology Single- or double-lumen Specialized right-angle needle is required to access the portal chamber. Located in subclavian vein; tip is located near the right atrium. "Power" Port may be used to inject contrast more quickly (e.g., for PE-protocol CT).	Long-term intravenous medications and/or fluids, especially chemotherapy Blood may be drawn from the catheter.	Intended for indefinite use
Tunneled cuffed catheters (Ash, DuraFlow, Tesio, etc.)	Dual-lumen catheters Placed by interventional radiology Can be placed in the internal jugular vein or subclavian vein	Used for hemodialysis Do not use catheter for any other reason without checking with the nephrologist.	Intermediate- to long-term use to allow graft or fistula maturation, if patients refuse permanent access, or if graft or fistula is contraindicated
Temporary hemodialysis catheters (Quinton, Trialysis)	Placed by nephrology or interventional radiology Nontunneled	Short-term hemodialysis Some types may also be used for medications or fluids (check with Nephrology first).	

Continued

TABLE 30-1 ALL YOU REALLY NEED TO KNOW ABOUT VASCULAR ACCESS—Cont'd

Type	Description	Common Uses	Duration of Use
Midline catheter	Kink proof material Peripherally placed by trained nursing personnel Located in antecubital vein Consider placement early before potential peripheral vessels are damaged.	Intermediate-term intravenous medications are planned (e.g., a several week course of antibiotics). Not intended for TPN or chemotherapy Blood drawing is discouraged (causes fibrin deposition at the tip and eventual catheter failure).	Intermediate-term use (1-6 wk) Heparin flushing should be performed when the catheter is not being used at least twice a day Can be removed at the bedside
PICC	17-inch catheter placed by trained nursing personnel Interventional radiology can place PICC lines under fluoroscopy if necessary Located in basilic, cephalic, or median cubital vein	Long-term intravenous medications are planned. TPN and more irritating medications may be given, provided the tip is in the superior vena cava Blood may be drawn from the catheter	Long-term use May be left in place indefinitely as long as functioning properly Can be removed at the bedside

Complications from catheter placement may include bleeding, pneumothorax, infection, and thrombosis. Some clotted catheters may be opened with alteplase (Cathflo, Activase). The various catheters require that specified amounts of the appropriately diluted solution be instilled to just fill the lumen, ensuring that the thrombolytic is not injected systemically. Your hospital will likely have specified procedures for declotting catheters, so do not attempt without knowing your local policy. Also, it may be advisable to check with the service that actually put the catheter in.
PE, pulmonary embolism; TPN, total parenteral nutrition; PICC, peripherally inserted central catheter.

Equipment

- This is in addition to what is typically needed for central venous access.
- A real-time 2D ultrasound machine with transducer: Make sure it is fully charged!
- Sterile plastic transducer sheath
- Sterile and nonsterile ultrasound gel (sterile gel is often included with the plastic transducer sheath kit)
- A nonsterile assistant is even more important when using ultrasound guidance.

Procedure

- First and foremost, track down and obtain a fully charged ultrasound machine.
- It is helpful to visualize the vascular structures at your access site prior to sterilization of the procedure site. This can be done with nonsterile ultrasound gel or surgical lubricant.
  - Note the depth and caliber of the vein.
  - Evaluate for vein patency and compressibility.
  - Identify adjacent structures. Remember, the vein is typically anterolateral to the artery for the IJ and medial to the artery for the femoral.
  - **Look for an alternate site if the vein is not well-visualized, if multiple collateral vessels without a single large lumen or if a central thrombus is visualized.**
- Cleanse and drape the patient; a full body drape is needed for central venous access.
- Apply sterile ultrasound gel to the interior of the plastic transducer sheath (alternatively, your nonsterile assistant may apply nonsterile gel to the ultrasound transducer).
- With the aid of your nonsterile assistant, carefully lower the ultrasound transducer into the opening of the plastic sheath (ensure that the transducer does not contact the outer surface of the sheath). The sheath should be pulled by the assistant to cover the length of the transducer cord that may contact the sterile field.
- Place sterile ultrasound gel on the patient at the selected access site.
- Once again locate the vein at the selected entry site. Rotate the ultrasound probe to obtain the transverse view (perpendicular to the course of the vein). As for the landmark technique, you should err initially on aiming your needle away from the artery

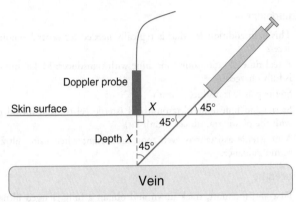

Figure 30-1. Needle insertion site using ultrasound guidance.

(e.g., laterally or toward the ipsilateral nipple for IJ access, and medially for femoral venous access). Before beginning, align your ultrasound view perpendicular to your intended needle path.

- After anesthetizing the area, insert your introducer needle from the central venous access kit at a 45° angle to the skin at a distance away from the transducer that is approximately equal to the depth of the vein (as previously measured [see Figure 30-1]). Assuming the vein is centered on the ultrasound screen, aim for the midpoint of the ultrasound probe with your needle. The needle will be visible on the ultrasound screen as it nears and enters the vessel. "Bouncing" the needle gently may allow for easier visualization of the tip of the needle. **When starting out, it is best to have a sterile assistant hold the ultrasound transducer for you to free both hands for the line placement.**

- Once venous return is obtained, the ultrasound probe may be left to the side on the sterile field.

- The other procedural aspects of central line placement are covered in detail on the accompanying procedure card.

OTHER PROCEDURES

All other procedures (i.e., arterial line placement, peripheral IV, thoracentesis, paracentesis, arthrocentesis, and lumbar puncture) are described in detail on the accompanying procedure card. Keep reading for details on using the ultrasound for thoracentesis and paracentesis.

Ultrasound for Thoracentesis

- Ultrasound should be used to visualize a pleural effusion and mark the site for thoracentesis. This has become standard of care, as studies have shown improved success rates and decreased complication rates with the use of ultrasound. A physical exam should still be performed to determine the extent of the effusion. Ultrasound is then used to visualize the effusion and mark the site for the procedure. Real-time ultrasound guidance (i.e., visualizing the effusion with the ultrasound probe while inserting the thoracentesis catheter) can be performed but is rarely necessary.

- To scan the chest with the ultrasound, ensure you are using the proper probe (a curvilinear or thoracic probe, NOT the vascular probe as this does not scan to the proper depth). Find someone who is skilled with the ultrasound to guide you. Scan for an area where several centimeters of fluid (will look black or anechoic) are superficial to the lung, also noting the location of the diaphragm and the depth of the effusion. Then mark the best site and proceed with the thoracentesis.

Ultrasound for Paracentesis

- Ultrasound may also be used to mark the site for paracentesis. The use of ultrasound likely improves success rates.

- Again, ensure that you are using the proper probe (same as for a thoracentesis).

- Scan the right and left lower quadrants, lateral to the inferior epigastric vessels, for a good pocket of fluid (again will look black or anechoic).

- Look for a site with at least several centimeters of fluid superficial to the bowel.

- The liver and spleen may be enlarged, so make note of these organs as well if visible on the screen.

- Mark the site and commence with the procedure.

- Real-time ultrasound guidance is rarely needed unless the fluid pocket is very small.

GUIDELINES FOR OCCUPATIONAL EXPOSURES

- If an exposure to blood or other bodily fluids occurs
  - **Stop what you are doing immediately**! Take a deep breath; don't panic.
  - Cleanse wound with soap and water. For mucous membrane exposures, rinse with copious amounts of water.

- Call the hospital's exposure hotline to report the exposure and get further instructions. **Each hospital has its own procedures on handling occupational exposures**; you likely heard about them in your orientation. Be sure to follow them. In reporting an incident, you will need the following information:
    - Date and time of exposure
    - Details of procedure being performed, amount of fluid or material exposed to, severity of exposure, type of needle used (e.g., hollow bore)
    - Details of exposure source—e.g., known HIV, hepatitis B virus (HBV), hepatitis c virus (HCV) positive? If source has known HIV, obtain the names and dosages of medications the source is taking.
  - You and the source patient will need to be evaluated for HIV, HBV, and HCV. Follow instructions from employee/occupational health for testing and follow-up.
- The risk of transmission of a blood-borne pathogen depends on the pathogen involved, the type of exposure, amount of blood involved in the exposure, and amount of virus in the patient's blood at the time of exposure.
- If you have been exposed, you should avoid exchange of bodily fluids with other persons until follow-up is complete, including using condoms with sexual partners until the results of the HIV test from the source patient are known.
- For more information on postexposure risk and therapies:
  - National Clinicians' Postexposure Hotline 1-888-448-4911 or http://nccc.ucsf.edu/clinician-consultation/pep-post-exposure-prophylaxis/ (last accessed July 6, 2017)
  - CDC https://www.cdc.gov/mmwr/PDF/rr/rr5011.pdf (last accessed July 6, 2017)

Final Thoughts

31

Thomas M. De Fer

1. Take primary responsibility for your patients—you are their doctor.

2. When in doubt, ask and ask again. Call someone (wake up someone if you need to), preferably someone who knows more than you do.

3. Stay organized and prioritize your tasks.

4. Real patient care first, documentation later.

5. When in doubt, it's always better (albeit more painful) to go and see the patient.

6. The right thing to do usually involves more time expenditure.

7. There is zero tolerance for making things up. If you don't know, you don't know. Say so. If it's important you'll remember next time.

8. Nurses are almost always right. If they are wrong, be selective about pointing this out.

9. Walk if you don't need to run. Sit down if you don't need to stand. Lie down if there's a bed nearby. Answer all of nature's calls. There is almost always time to refuel (i.e., eat).

10. Listen to your patients. They'll usually tell you what you need to know.

11. Resist the temptation to discuss patient care in public areas; no good can come of it.

12. A healthy amount of compassion and compulsion makes it difficult to harm patients.

13. See one, do one, teach one. You'll be expected to assume more teaching responsibilities as time goes on. Start developing your own teaching style and discuss expectations clearly with all learners. You already know way more than you think.

14. Be really selective about your battles. If it won't help your patient, it's probably not worth it. Even at that, bad behavior will be remembered, and not in a good way.

15. Help out your colleagues. If you finish your work early, check with other members of your team or cross-covering interns to see if they need anything; they can return the favor when you need it most.

16. Before going home for the day, make sure your patients are tucked in and check out with your resident. A complete and clear sign-out is vital—make sure to include any information (studies, consultations, procedures) that may be needed to make major therapeutic decisions (see "Handoffs" section in Chapter 8, Daily Assessments).

17. Worthy goals for internship include learning to distinguish the life-threatening issues from the acute ones and from the stable ones; improving your ability to communicate in difficult situations; mastering the interpretation and proper usage of diagnostic tests; learning procedural skills; refining the ability to ask specific questions for every consultation you request.

18. Fear and anxiety are normal. Take a deep breath and plunge in—there are people around to help you. If you are feeling overwhelmed by fear, anxiety, or other emotions, seek help—don't be a hero!

19. There is no magic spell on the last day of internship that will turn you into a resident. Trust that if you do and learn the right things during internship, you will be prepared to rise to the challenges of residency.

20. And remember, "Intern year is only a year!" It will go much faster than you think, and you'll have much more fun than you think.

Index

Note: Page numbers followed by "f" indicate figures and "t" indicate tables.